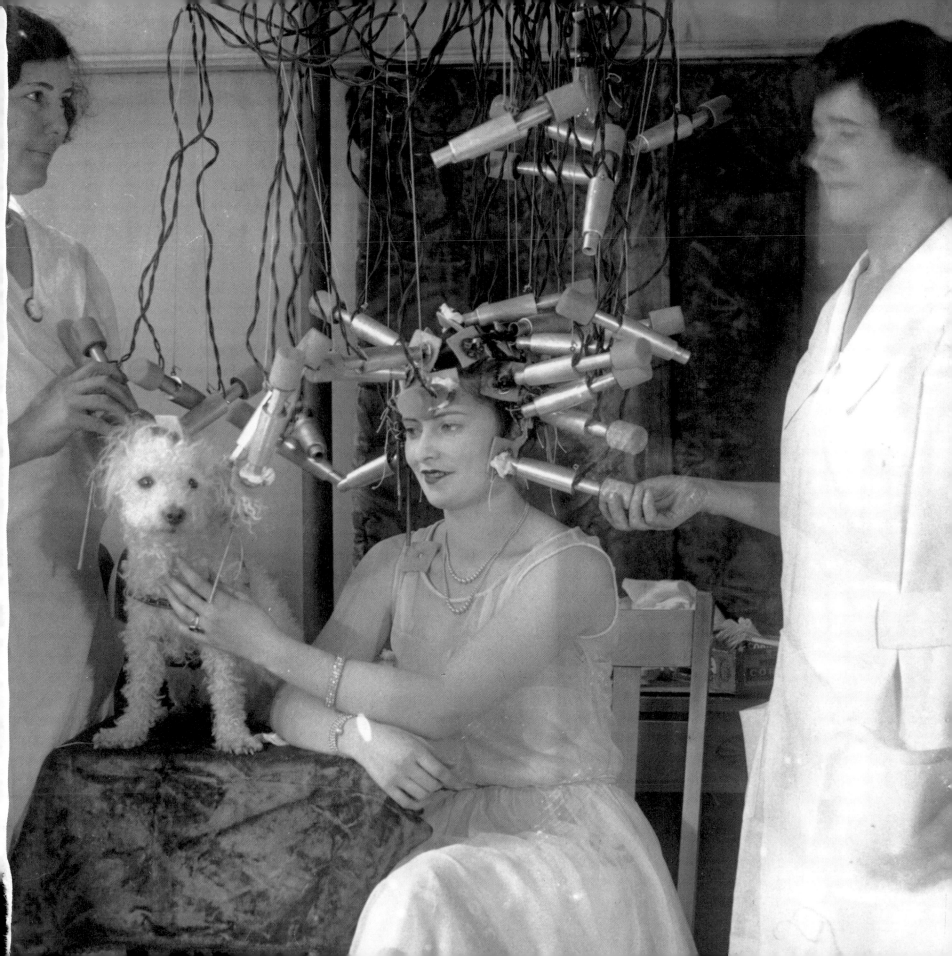

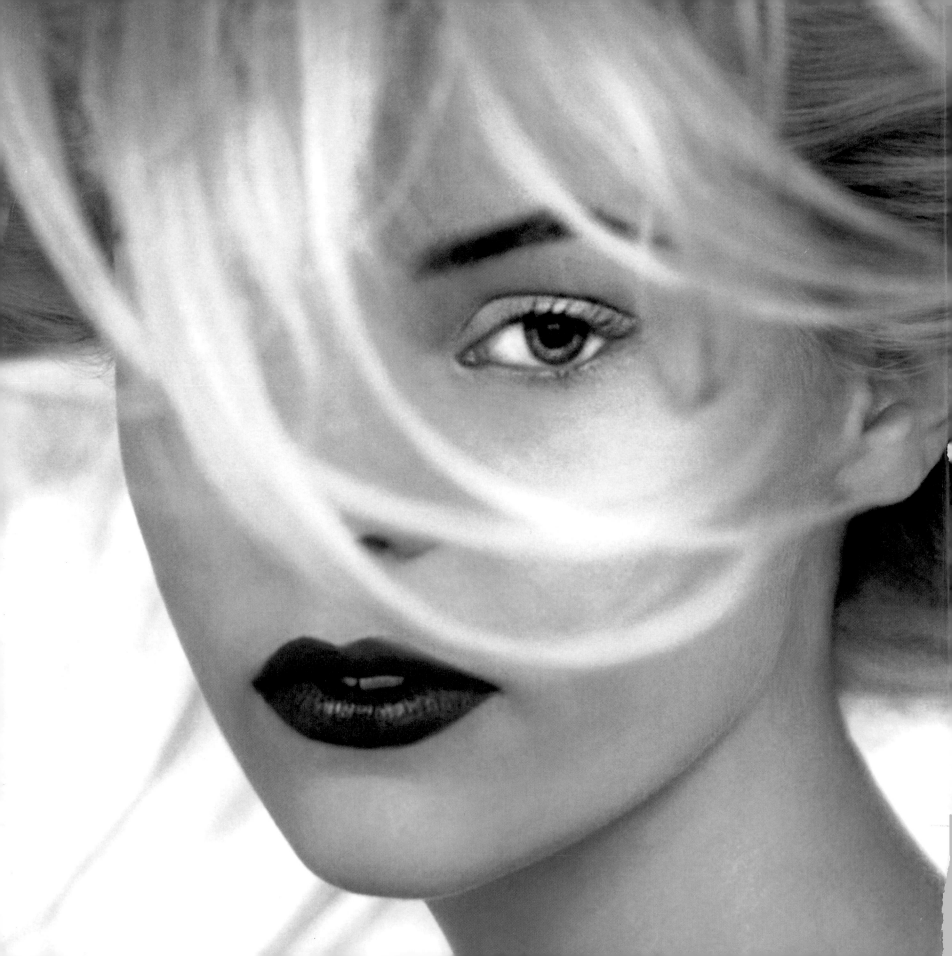

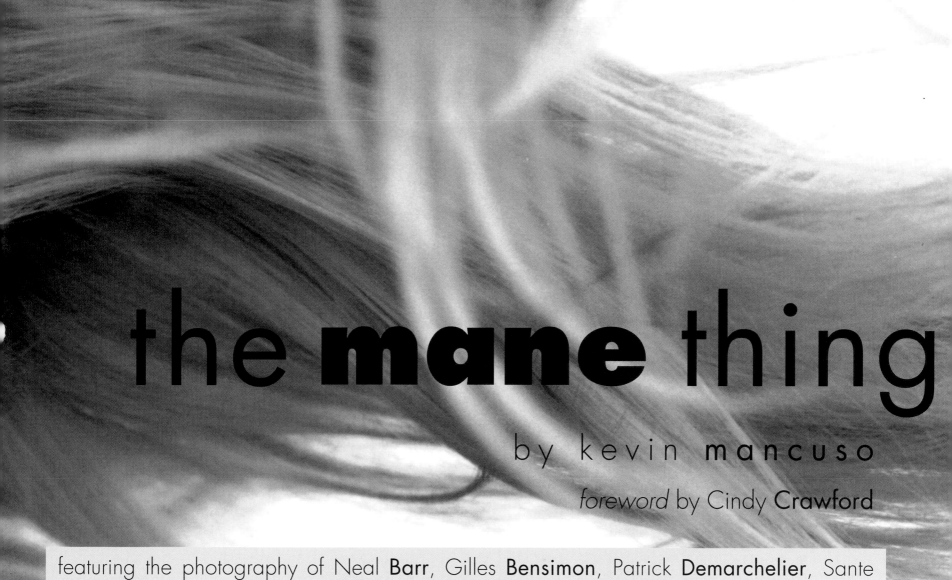

the **mane** thing

by kevin mancuso

foreword by Cindy Crawford

featuring the photography of Neal **Barr**, Gilles **Bensimon**, Patrick **Demarchelier**, Sante **D'Orazio**, Arthur **Elgort**, Don **Flood**, Nicolai **Grosell**, Torkil **Gudnason**, George **Holz**, Marc **Hom**, Wayne **Maser**, Matthew **Rolston**, Francesco **Scavullo**, Mark **Seliger**, Patric **Shaw**, Troy **Word**, and Jay **Zukerkorn**

creative direction, design, and illustrations by Donald F. Reuter

Little, Brown and Company • Boston • New York • London

First Edition

Library of Congress Cataloging-in-Publication Data

Mancuso, Kevin.
   The mane thing / Kevin Mancuso. — 1st ed.
        p.   cm.
     ISBN 0–316–16614–6
     1. Hairdressing. 2. Hairstyles. 3. Haircutting. I. Title.
TT972.M25   1999
   646.7'24 — dc21   98–49591

10 9 8 7 6 5 4 3 2 1

RRD–OH

Printed in the United States of America

Visit Kevin Mancuso's web site at **www.the-mane-thing.com**

~ opening page: During the twenties, machine technology hadn't quite kept up with the popularity of getting a hair permanent. This left women to be subjected to a torturous and arduous ordeal, one that was often quite dangerous, too. The "perming machine" was an archaic contraption that consisted mainly of heated rods suspended from overhead, which were clamped onto the subject's tender hair. In this memorable picture we see socialite Mrs. Agnes O'Laughlin and her dog merrily awaiting the outcome of a day of beauty, along with two salon technicians. Photo courtesy of UPI/Corbis-Bettmann.

~ preceding spread: Fabulous model James King has a superabundance of beautiful blond hair, here being shown to great effect with the use of a handheld fan. Photographed by Don Flood.

~ to the right: Beautiful Kashanna Evans has that ever rarer occurrence, a natural afro. Believe me, just to maintain it at this incredible length is no easy accomplishment. And to prove what a change your hair can make to your appearance, when she arrived on the set neither I nor photographer Neal Barr recognized her, even though the last time we both saw her was only a few months before. But then her hair had been blown out straight, and she looked totally different.

This book is dedicated to Rory Bernal, the first person I worked with in the business and my best friend. I miss you and wish you were here to share this with me.

Kashanna Evans, photographed by Neal Barr

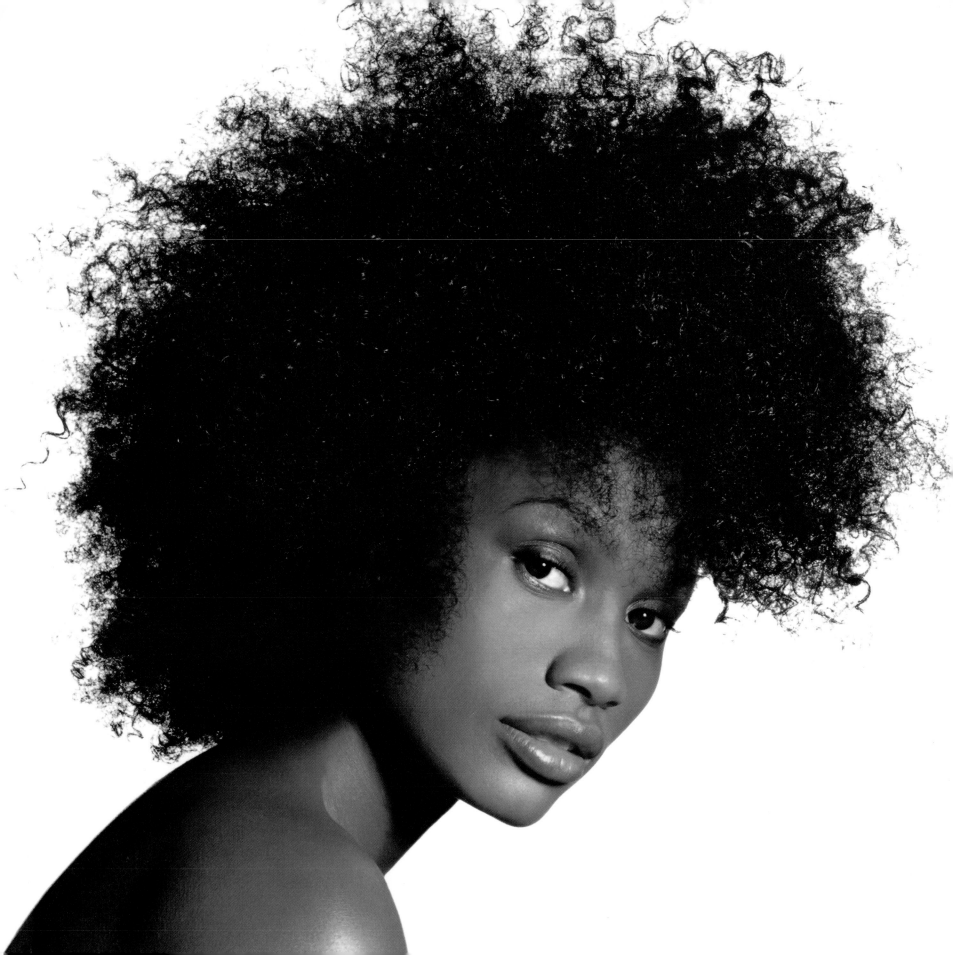

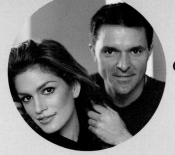
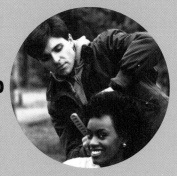
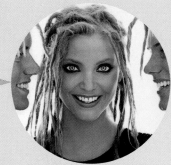
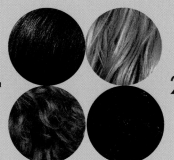
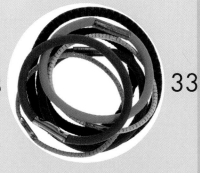
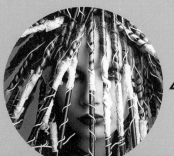

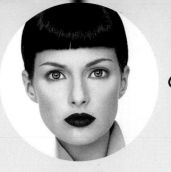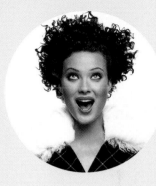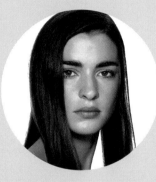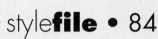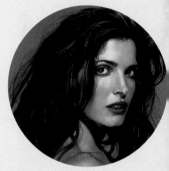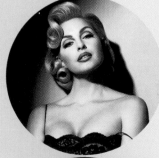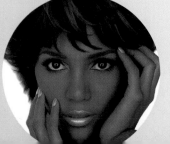

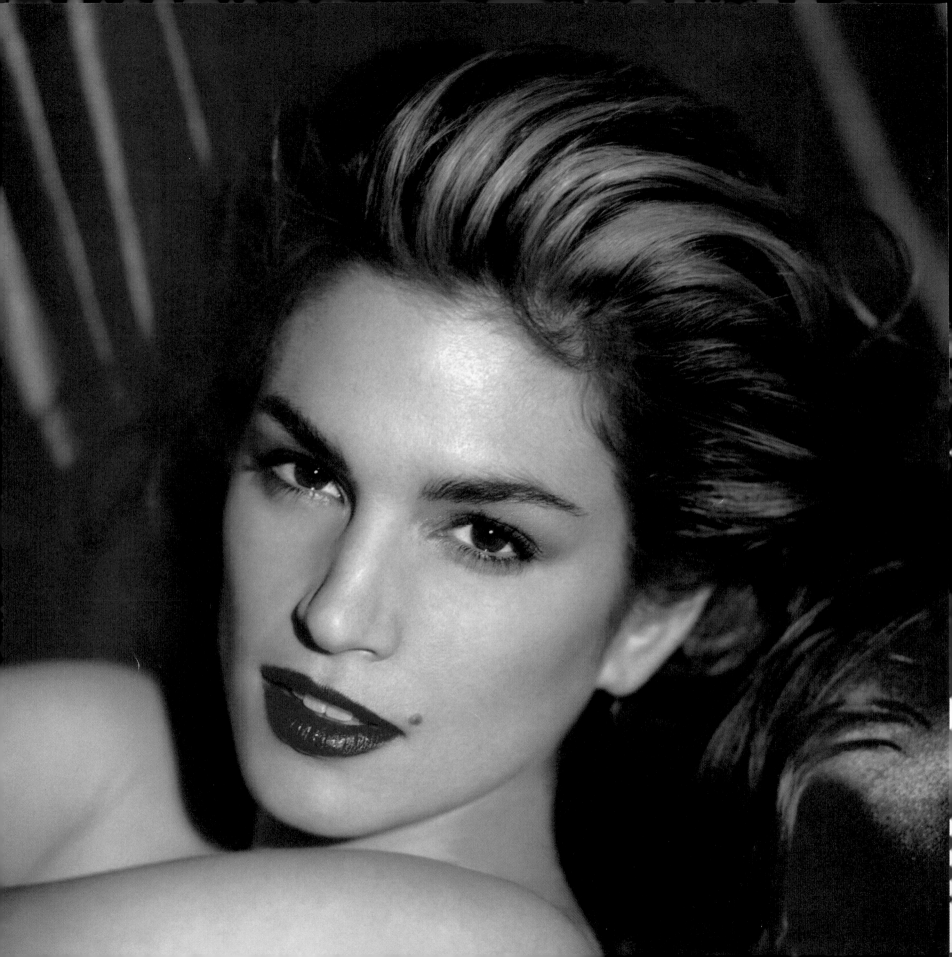

Can I just start out by saying how proud I am of my friend Kevin for doing this book? Having dabbled in the literary world myself (yes, that is a joke), I do know how much goes into actually putting a book together—clearing the photos, arranging the shoots, doing the writing, selling the concept, not to mention meeting after meeting. Hooray, Kevin—you've done it. This kind of thing is really the best part of where I am in my career—watching my friends (and myself) grow up and do our own thing.

I've been working with Kevin for years. In fact, we started working together pretty much at the beginning of my introduction to the "fabulous world of fashion." One spring night, over dinner at my house, we were discussing this foreword and I asked him if he remembered when we first met. We're not 100% sure, but we think it was at Eric Bowman's studio, where we were shooting an ad for some eyewear campaign. Kevin's memory is clearer about this day than mine. Here's why: He had set my hair in Velcro rollers and was going for that eighties "bigger-is-better" look (that I still can't help loving). Apparently, it was a typical New York City summer day—95 degrees and *lots* of humidity. Unfortunately, there was no air-conditioning in the studio and all that hot, muggy air was blowing through the windows and into my hair. Well, as if you didn't already know, hair and humidity don't mix, and Kevin

fore**word**

lucky lady This portrait (one of my favorites) was actually the last shot of a long day of shooting. Basically, Cindy just wanted to lie down. The fact that her hair (and makeup) still looked great after countless pictures, combined with the warm amber glow of the late-day sun, created one of those moments that make the work worth it all. Fab photog Sante D'Orazio captured it so perfectly the picture ended up on the cover of Spanish *Vogue*.

was, understandably, quite frustrated. Nothing he did could keep the curl or fullness in my hair. Our first job together turned out to be a disaster. It just goes to show you that even hair magicians like Kevin Mancuso have bad hair days—even if it's not their hair!

Cut to over a decade later. I've done more jobs that I can remember with Kevin. Everything from magazine covers (*Cosmopolitan*, *Allure*, *Vogue*, et al.) to Revlon ads. I love working with Kevin for two reasons. One, he's extremely funny, and we always laugh and laugh and laugh, and that makes the day just slip by. Two, I totally trust his sense of style and technique, and believe me, that takes a lot off my mind. My hair is literally putty in his hands.

I'm sure you could figure out on your own that I'm a bit picky about my hair. Professionally, it is a big part of my trademark. That's why it's crucial that it look right and that I feel good about it. I'm a girl (okay, maybe at thirty-two that's pushing it) and I want my hair to feel sexy and pretty, and for my husband to be able to get his hands through it. One of the advantages to my line of work is the chance to work with the most gifted artists in the business, and I do mean artists. And if you have half a brain (and that isn't saying we all do), you can't help but pick up a thing or two—even if it's just by osmosis. (Two hours in hair and makeup is a lot of time to read "Page Six.") One of the many things I've learned from Kevin is understanding how important the *texture* of hair is. For him, hairstyles come and go, but the basis of hair care is all about *texture*. First thing in the morning, he'll take his time with my hair, layering in the texture with different products and appliances. Once the texture is set, my hair looks great all day—even if I'm outside, in front of a wind fan, or flipping my head up and down for those hair commercials you've probably seen. Now I know it might sound a bit complicated or radical not talking in terms of "beehives," "shags," or "pageboys," but relax, Kevin's going to walk you right through it. And it won't hurt a bit.

Kevin, thanks for all the great times and for giving such good head! I love you!

Cindy
October 1998

easy does it
Photographer Arthur Elgort excels in, among other things, effortlessly capturing a subject's *natural* beauty. The wonderfully nonhectic mood around his set helps, too. Put Cindy in this equation, and a day of shooting can feel just like hanging out with your best friends. The only difference is you get some great pictures that end up as a spread in British *Vogue*.

Cindy Crawford, photographed by Arthur Elgort for British Vogue

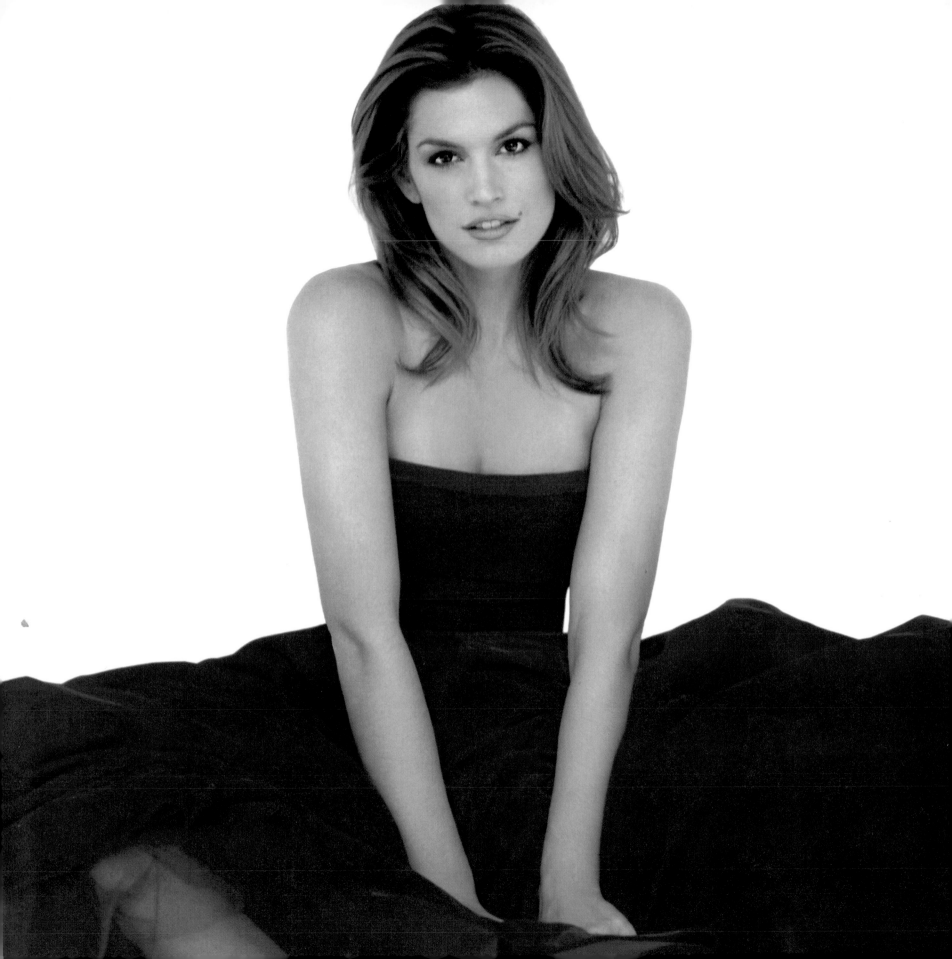

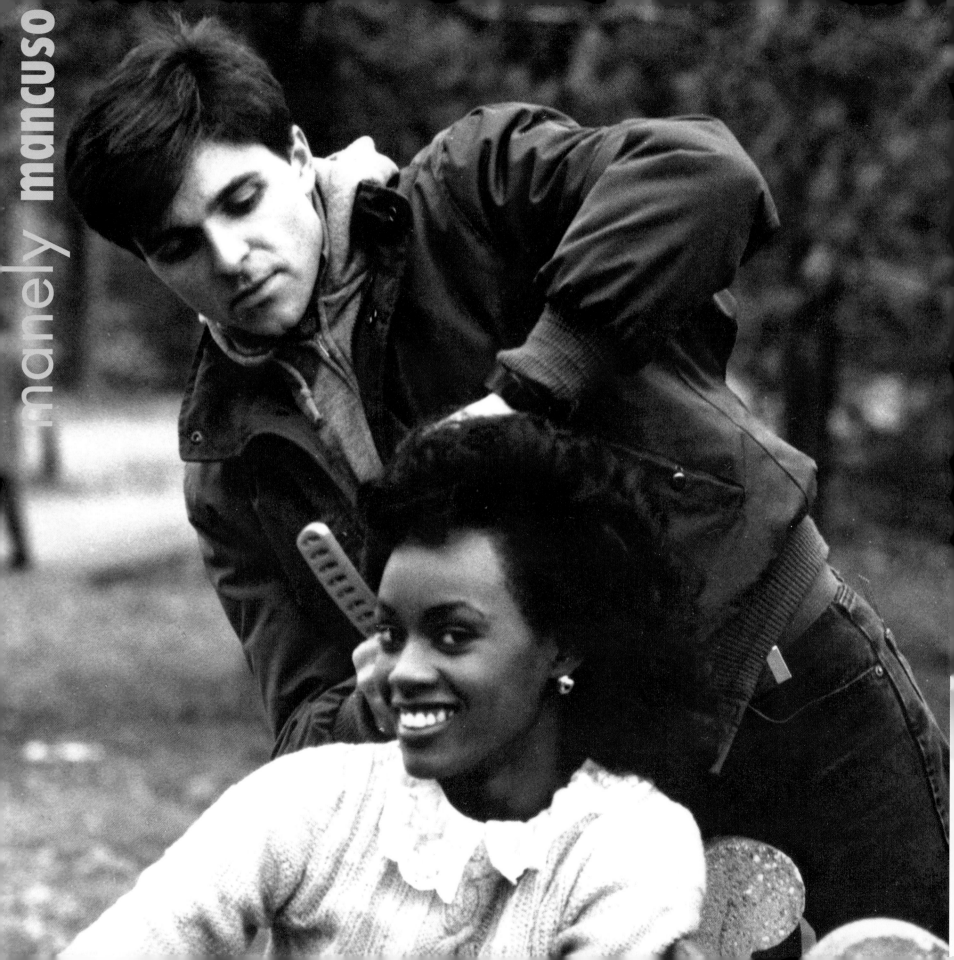

manely mancuso

My most vivid memories of early childhood involve the color of women's hair. In Brooklyn and Staten Island (where I was brought up) hair came in all different shades of the rainbow—from apricot to rust, blue rinses to purple grays, and every once in a while I'd see a double-process blond, looking way too yellow. The hairdos, to me, often resembled food, like artichokes and cotton candy. There was even the one that looked just like a bag of Jiffy Pop (you know, when the container is all puffed up from being heated right before you rip open the foil). All very curious and interesting looks, especially to a kid.

When I wasn't wreaking havoc with my neighborhood friends, I would spend time watching and admiring the ease and enjoyment with which the women around me, especially my mother, combined tending the house, cooking the family meals, and, of all things, styling their own hair. From my earliest recollections, my mom doted on her hair, and to this day she will color and set it herself. (On one occasion, she attempted a home perm with disastrous results. A few days before my sister's wedding she tried one, and all her hair broke off. Those of you at home—be careful.) She was also quite inventive when it came to the techniques she used to create some rather amazing styles. Think about coming home from school to find your mother with her wet hair all twisted and knotted up with pipe cleaners, looking like Buckwheat meets Burnett (Carol, that is) and

singing Jeanette MacDonald songs as she prepared spaghetti and meatballs. Imagine the family's astonishment as she emerged from the bathroom a few hours later with the most spectacular Lana Turnerish, Betty Grablesque, showstopping coif. Other times, if the mood hit her, we'd be treated to a devastating Marilyn Monroe flip or her version of the infamous "astronaut's wife" look (otherwise referred to as "helmet hair"). This lasted well into my adolescence, with mom dazzling us with her unending parade of derring-dos. As far as my wanting to be a hairstylist, I guess you could say it was genetically determined!

When I was a young teen, I was into that David Bowie–Rod Stewart glam rock thing that all the cool kids were into at the time. The family was now living in New Jersey, and I was attending, of all things, a vocational high school that specialized in classes in auto mechanics and construction. At home, even though my brothers and I would help Dad with landscaping the yard and refinishing the house, I did not enjoy wiring the walls and soldering pipes. And as far as school was concerned, I couldn't stand those do-it-yourself-type classes. My alternative was a course called "Distributive Education" (I still have no idea what that means), which consisted of selling in the

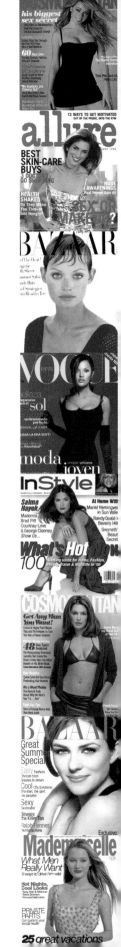

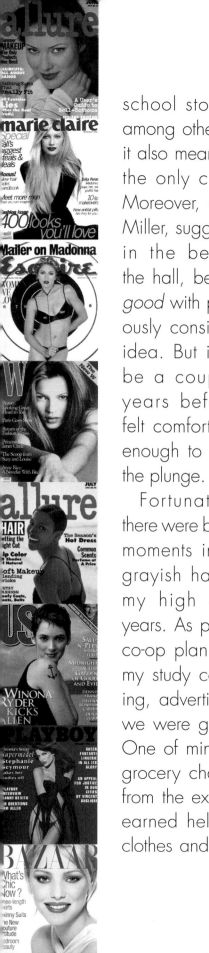

school store and decorating windows, among other equally taxing activities. What it also meant was that I ended up in one of the only classes that had girls in them. Moreover, at one point my instructor, Mrs. Miller, suggested that I think about enrolling in the beauty course down the hall, because I was so *good* with people. I seriously considered the idea. But it would be a couple of years before I felt comfortable enough to take the plunge.

Fortunately, there were bright moments in the grayish haze of my high school years. As part of the co-op plan for one of my study courses (marketing, advertising, and display), we were given jobs in related fields. One of mine was as a part-time clerk at a grocery chain. I can't say I learned much from the experience, but the extra income I earned helped keep me in some groovy clothes and allowed me to indulge in some

very expensive haircuts for the time. (Can you imagine a teen caring enough back in the early seventies to get his hair clipped for thirty-five to sixty-five dollars a pop?) Once I finally graduated, I went to work in a barbeque grill factory, and during the weekends I would hang out with friends who had formed their own band. At that time I was studying sound engineering at Electric Lady Studio in Greenwich Village, and I would have stayed in the area if the education part hadn't been so expensive. Instead I took what was left of my earnings, combined with a welfare check and some food stamps (times were hard), and moved with a friend to a fourth-floor walk-up on the Upper East Side of Manhattan. By taking a weekend job at an after-hours club I managed to have just enough money left over every month to take that fateful first step and finally enroll in a beauty school.

I have to say the reality of the required thousand hours of beauty school was not all that I had hoped it would be. I ended up learning more from practical experience and outside opportunities.

14

Elizabeth Hurley, photographed by Torkil Gudnason for Estée Lauder

And in this regard I may have been luckier than other students. My roommate at the time, Willie Chu, was working as an assistant for photographer Ara Gallant (who had himself begun years before as a hairstylist), and on many occasions I would accompany him to shoots. I loved it! There was always some model like Janice Dickenson, Iman, or Apollonia being photographed for Italian *Vogue* or *Interview,* and Ara's amazing work and tutelage became major influences on my career. I would assist around the set and eventually started doing hair myself when another good friend, Rory, was booked. Rory was a hair and makeup artist who, along with his companion Fernando, worked out of an Act II salon. On my off-hours from school I worked with them and learned how to relax, straighten, perm, and double process hair better than I did in any of my classes. Upon graduation, I continued on at Act II. Then, in the summer of 1980, I went to work as an apprentice stylist at Vidal Sassoon. The place was like precision-haircutting boot camp, but it was fantastic.

How could it not be? It was the time when the new-wave group Flock of Seagulls, with their wild hairstyles, and the "wedge" cut were at the peak of their popularity.

The following summer, I moved on to the John Dellaria salon. John is considered a hairstylist's stylist, and working there was quite interesting coming on the heels of Sassoon, because John specialized in a sort of *anti*-precision haircut (he would give someone a cut that looked like a bob in front and surprise you with something like a hair explosion in the back). I stayed there through the mid-eighties, becoming his top stylist and creative director (basically in charge of the image of the salon and teaching the stylists all the latest techniques and cuts).

Then, by late 1985, I became part of a hairstyling revolution of my own. I and fellow Dellaria stylists Danilo and Oribe,

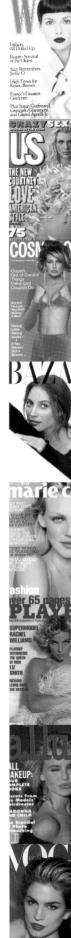

Nona Hendryx, photographed by Geoffrey Thomas

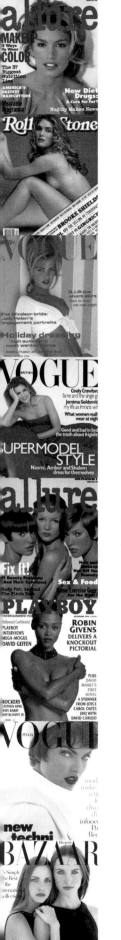

joined by Eric Gabriel and Losi, jumped ship and started the salon Oribe at Parachute. At the time, Oribe's partner, Omar, asked me if I was interested in taking on managerial and educational duties similar to the ones I had done for John in this new venture; I jumped at the chance. It was the beginning of the ascent for all of us into the fashion limelight. My own really came about after a good friend, editor Paul Cavaco, introduced me to photographer Eric Bowman—yes, of *that* Cindy Crawford shoot; amazingly, Eric booked me immediately the next day for the start of a series of German *Vogue* covers, which ended up including supermodels Linda Evangelista, Paulina Porizkova, and Stephanie Seymour. (I guess the pictures of Cindy didn't turn out quite as bad as I thought).

I stayed with Oribe and crew right up to 1990, then left and went to Pierre Michel (at the Plaza). Finally, in 1992, I opened up with the Peter Coppola salon (again as creative director). In addition, I maintain an editorial and advertising schedule that allows me to work with a loyal following of clients, and I see new ones on a regular basis. (Even though it may seem like stylists move around quite a bit, in this business mobility is a part of the game; it keeps you fresh with new ideas.)

In the last few years, I began to compile and write down all the techniques I have used throughout my professional career. (This became necessary while doing a stint as cyber-editor for *American Salon* magazine and working as resident hair guru on the Lifetime show *Wired*.) Once I had all the materials collected, it dawned on me that they might make a book. Personally and professionally, I was frustrated by the lack of what I considered accessible and interesting information on the field of hairstyling. So I made it a point to gather everything together and combine it in an attractive and interesting format, expecting to accomplish that very thing. I hope I've succeeded. However, the bottom line is not whether I have pleased myself, but if I am able to get you to understand and enjoy the ongoing processes of styling and living with your hair.

a bit of hair-story *page 12*: This shot was taken "behind the scenes" at one of my very first jobs (at least twenty years ago, yikes!). It was outside in Central Park, New York, and the temperature was about thirty degrees. How the model could keep smiling was beyond me.
page 14: One of many times I have worked with gorgeous Elizabeth Hurley (this was for Estée Lauder, taken by Torkil Gudnason). By the way, this is the second hairstyle done that day. Turn to page 114 to see the first.
page 15: Legendary songstress Nona Hendryx, who started out as a customer of mine at John Dellaria and ended up as one of my closest friends. Much of the style was done using temporary hair extensions.
to the right: A lighthearted moment, backstage at a Donna Karan runway show. Photograph by Michel Arnaud.
along the edges: A gathering of some of my favorite magazine covers.

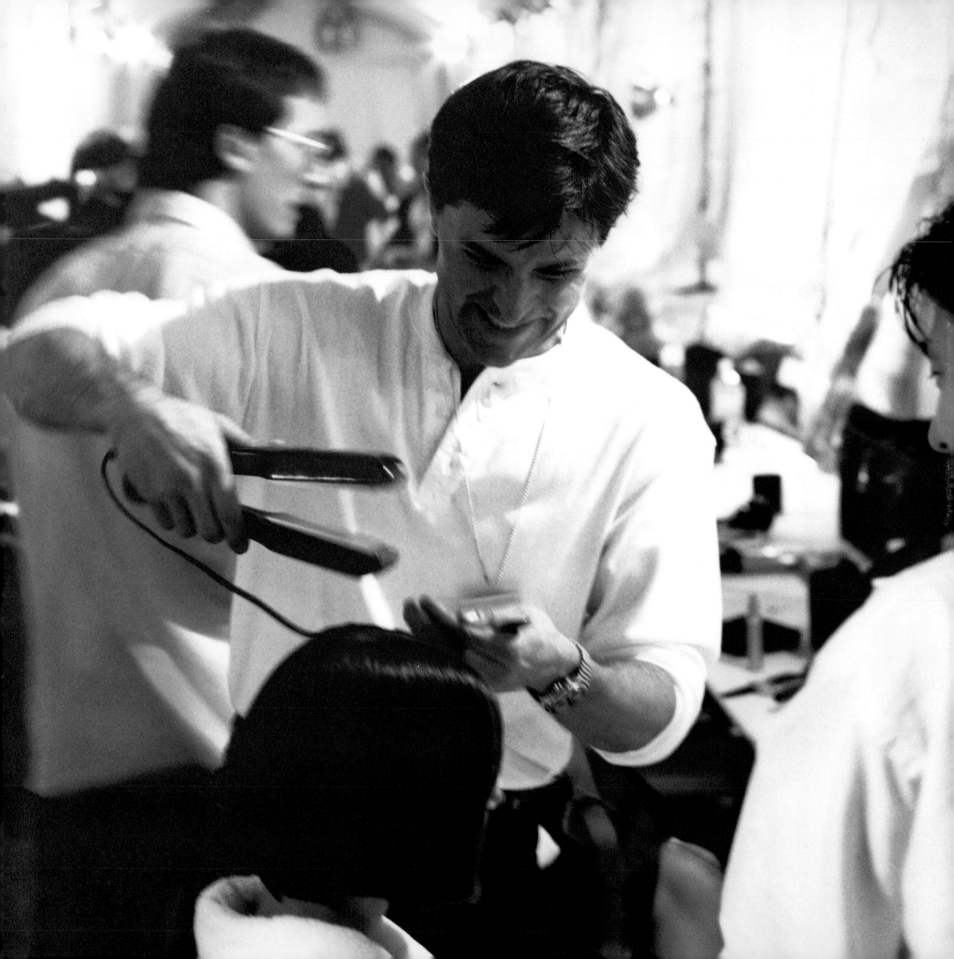

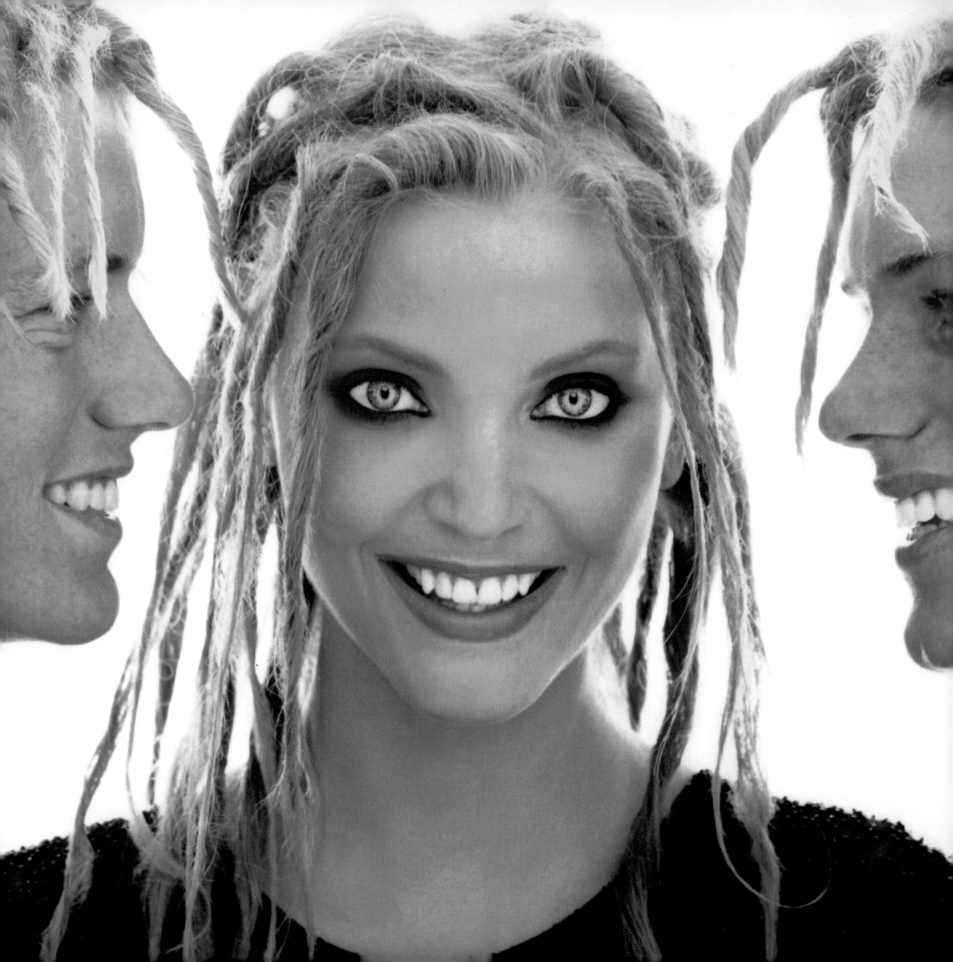

Here is something I want you to consider the next time you think about your hair: The images you see in magazines, in movies, and on television are something of a fiction. At the very minimum, there are at least five people behind every editorial photo of a model—the photographer, his or her assistants, the makeup artist, the clothing stylist, maybe a manicurist, not to mention the studio personnel, maybe a prop person, the people back at the magazine, and, of course, the hairstylist, and oh! don't forget the retoucher—and usually twice (sometimes even five to ten times) that for every commercial. And if you have more than one model or actress, these numbers can more than double. If you take into account how your hair behaves and looks normally, even under the best of circumstances, you begin to see the large discrepancy between fantasy (basically, all the above media images) and reality. I bring this point up not to deride a business that I am very proud and excited to be a part of, just to clarify that these images are meant to provoke and inspire us. And in order for them to do that, some liberties must be taken. But as far as I am concerned, they are never created intentionally to cause anxiety or disappointment with what you have.

Fortunately, most people do not look at hair and hairstyles in the same way they once did. It used to be that you would have your hair cut and configured into the latest version of a favorite celebrity's hair, regardless of whether or not the look really suited you or your hair. (The

~ To get this Rasta-inspired look on all three models took a lot of time and patience, but it wasn't really that hard to do. I just grouped the hair into sections (about one inch wide each) and started twisting and back combing. It's totally bad for your hair, but so much fun. Just hope you're not the one left combing it out!

locktalk

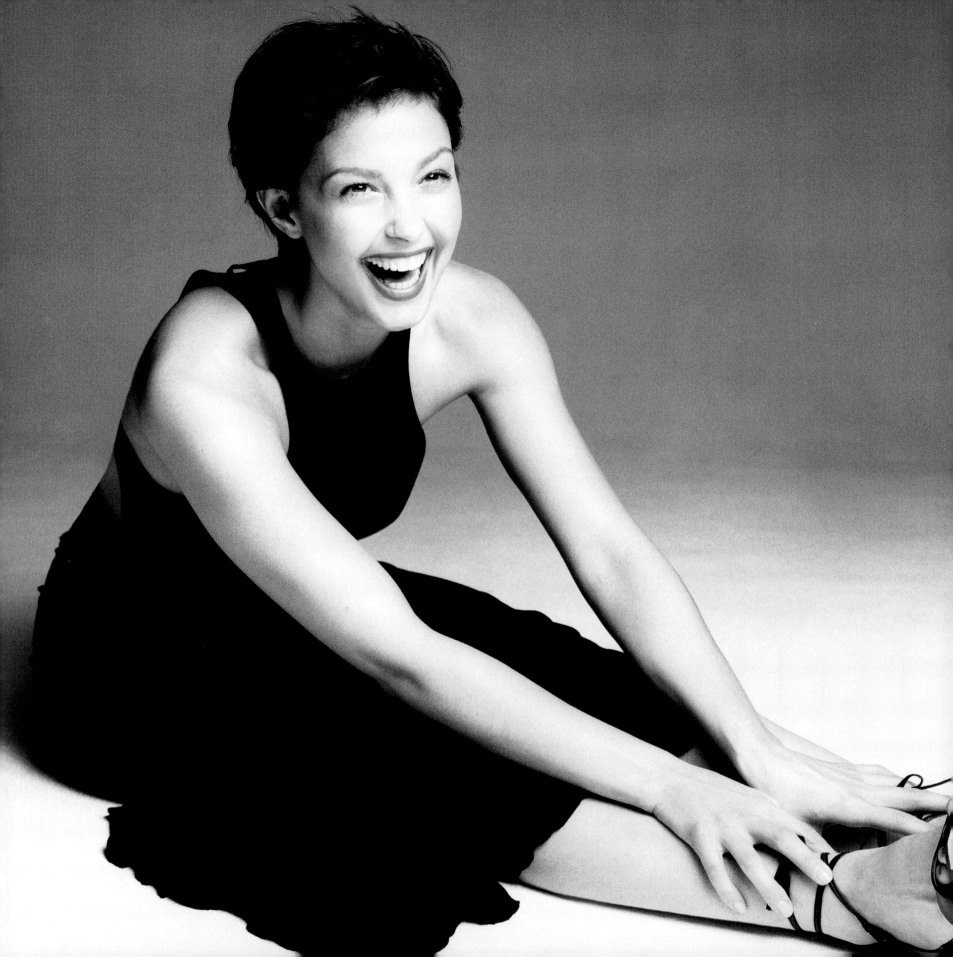

~ They say one picture is worth a thousand words. Well, how about two? Ashley Judd is one of those women with whom I have had the pleasure to work on numerous occasions who can go from one extreme of the beauty spectrum to the other and come out looking stunning either way. Here, she's sporting a short, natural cut. Adorable. Now turn to page 141 for a look at her with bleach-blond locks. A knockout in any guise.

fact that you might not be able to successfully re-create it on your own was also cause for much more unhappiness than the situation called for.) Thankfully, this does not go on anymore, or at least not in the same way. Sure, you may want to look like Cindy Crawford or Halle Berry, but you're looking to re-create a *mood* more than an exact duplication of the hairstyle itself. In general, that's because hairstyling now takes into consideration the importance of hair texture, both literally and figuratively. We are now going for both a look *and* a feel with our hair at the same time. Furthermore, there is a better understanding of the limitations *and* possibilities inherent in each different texture (from rough to smooth and everything in between), and that knowledge is the key to styling (and living with) our hair successfully. With a little care, consideration, and information, the choices are far more abundant than we once thought.

By writing and putting together this book, I hope to tear down the mystique surrounding hair (creating the illusion that only a chosen few know its cherished secrets) and show you how easy it is to take care of and work with. Since I can't consult with each and every one of you individually, I have tried to make the information as *generally* helpful as possible. Presented in the form of a workbook (or even a cookbook), the steps are all laid out for you. All you have to do is follow along, adding an extra dash of this here and maybe not putting in so much of that there (of course, according to your individual hair type and needs), and only if the mood suits you. I hope that by the time you reach the end, you'll understand that successful individual hair care is not about a handful of magician's tricks and that the power to control unruly, unmanageable, or unworkable hair was there all along, waiting for you to take charge.

Ashley Judd, photographed by Patrick Demarchelier for Harper's Bazaar

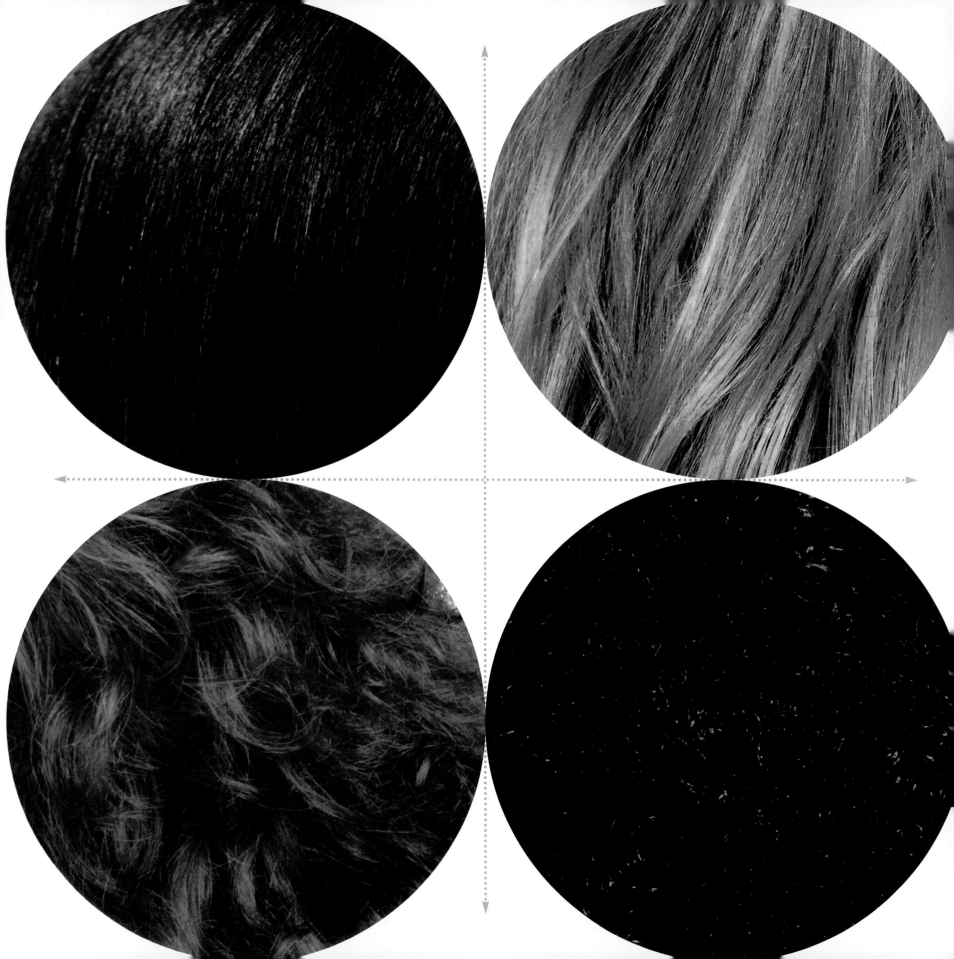

What is the one thing you notice when you meet people for the very first time? As you might guess, I notice their hair. In fact, within a matter of seconds, I will have taken into account whether their hair is in good condition or bad, if the style is right for them, if the color is natural, and so on. However, even though you might have said something like the eyes, I wouldn't be surprised if you hadn't already taken for granted that the person had a nice head of hair. Now why is this? My feeling is that what great hair does best for a person may be more subliminal than overt. Really good hair acts like the frame on a beautiful painting, not overwhelming or upstaging the artistry it surrounds.

But in order to "frame" your looks successfully, you need to know what you're dealing with and how best to work with what you've got. In this chapter I'm going to give you some basic facts about your hair. However, I must qualify a few things before we get started. For one, I do not want to be presumptuous about anything or make gross generalizations about your hair. In addition, throughout the book I have made an effort not to be stereotypical in how I represent different types of beauty (and how hair should be worn by any ethnic type). However, the four women I use to illustrate the basic hair types (straight, wavy, curly, and kinky) in this chapter do fit a preconcieved mold. My thought was that in order to impart the most information in the least amount of space, I should give people what they expect to see, but acknowledge that no one individual necessarily fits exactly into a single category.

~ clockwise, from top left: the four basic hair groups— straight, wavy, kinky, and curly.

hair
apparent

curly

Isn't it interesting that so many people with curly hair want straight hair and will do whatever it takes to get it? Curly hair is high maintenance: Most curly textures have a natural coarseness, making hair feel and appear dry; the hair becomes dehydrated, making the daily styling routine more work than for those with straight hair. Curly textures frizz, bend, and curl in humidity, sometimes uncontrollably. Overall, with curly hair it is hard to control the volume and definition of the hair. Also be aware that chemical processes (perming, coloring, bleaching, etc.) can take the definition out of curly hair and leave it frizzy. However, what curly hair has aplenty is versatility. Where straight hair might need product texturizing to give it volume and pliability, curly hair has this naturally, allowing for the freedom to create many styles, especially anything up, like an up-twist, ponytails, or looks requiring pins or decoration in the hair. For the most part, too, it straightens easily and because of its natural configuration, takes to shapely styles with great ease.

kinky

This describes a wide variety of configurations—frizzy, spiralled, mixed frizzy, and textured curl—all within a range of textures, from very fine to very thick. It is also sometimes the most fragile of all hair types, prone to damage and breaking, because it has the fewest cuticle layers (which hold individual hair strands together). Chemical treatments can cause problems if not handled with great care. However, kinky hair benefits from conditioning, relaxes and straightens easily, and can hold curly styles with great success. It also has a fantastic sheen, which can be enhanced with suitable styling aids. Kinky hair is also "self-supportive." What this means is that in its naturally dry (unrelaxed) state, it can be fashioned into

shapes, like the one on model Kashanna Evans to the right, and hold the style with relative ease and not need spraying. Another important characteristic to frizzy, coarse hair is that it normally grows very dense and can trap oil and dead skin against the scalp, making it important to properly cleanse it on a regular basis, regardless of whether or not your hair is exceptionally dry or coarse.

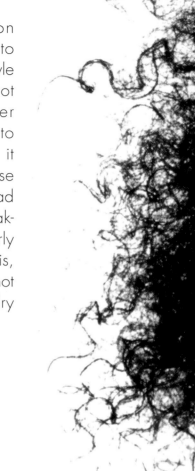

~ *Because both curly hair (see Heather Dillon on page 26) and kinky hair (to the right, on Kashanna Evans) are prone to dehydration, it is always a good idea to condition it, especially if you keep it longer (the farther hair grows from the scalp, the more damage can occur).*

Kashanna Evans, photographed by Neal Barr

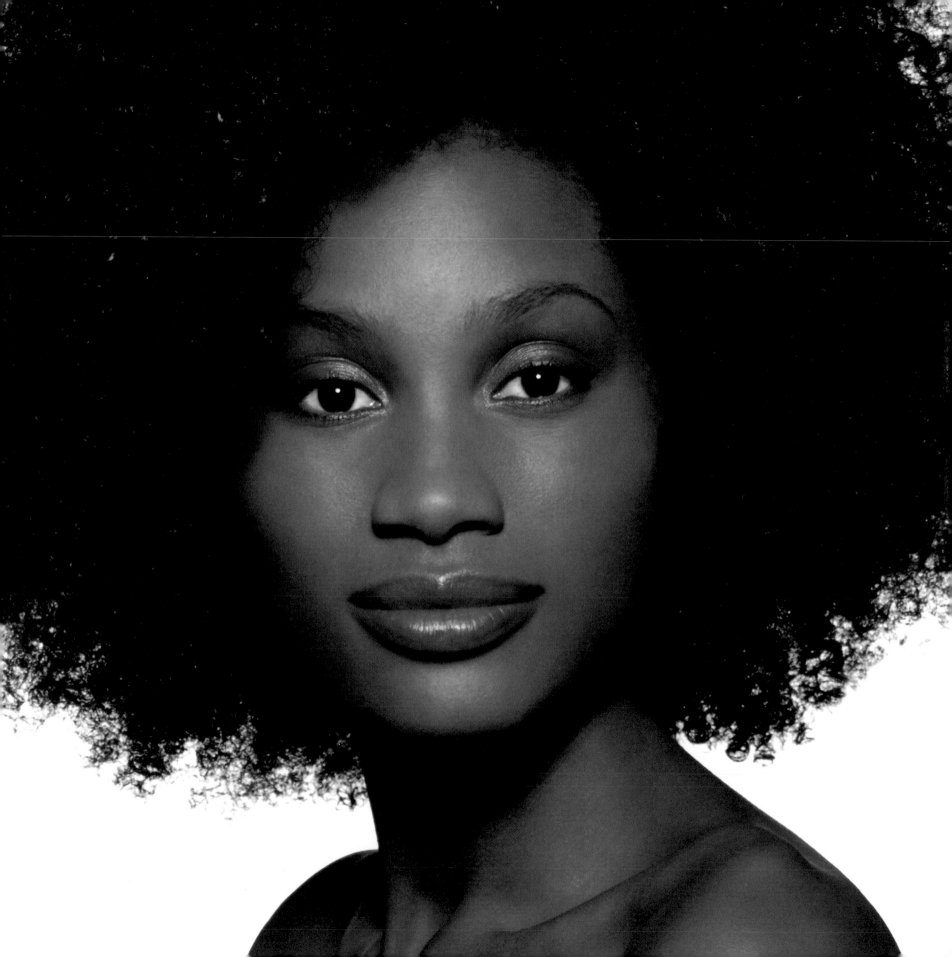

the **root** of things

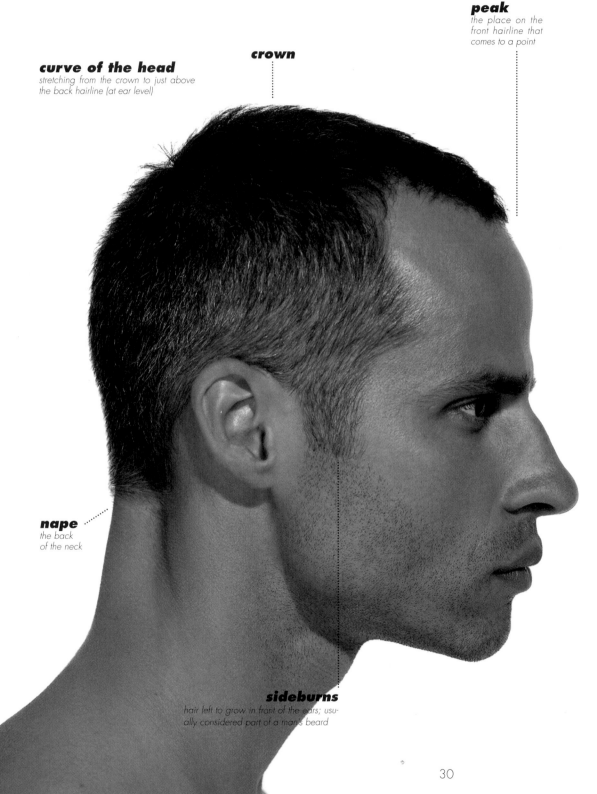

curve of the head
stretching from the crown to just above the back hairline (at ear level)

crown

peak
the place on the front hairline that comes to a point

nape
the back of the neck

sideburns
hair left to grow in front of the ears; usually considered part of a man's beard

At any given moment a person will have approximately 100 to 120,000 individual hairs on his or her head. (Interestingly, blonds have the most hair and redheads have the least.)

An individual hair follicle (or shaft) is made up of two parts: the outer cuticle layer, which serves as protection for the inner—cortex and medulla—layer. Be aware that the cuticle layer is the one most affected by your everyday routine. If it is damaged, it will show. However, the inner support layer can also be altered by a number of chemical processes.

The hair follicle is only alive at the point where it is rooted in your scalp. From there the keratin (a protein substance) that is pushed to the surface is dead. Alongside each hair root is a sebaceous gland; this is the one that produces those oily secretions. Then there is a sweat gland, plenty of blood vessels (for nourishment), and even a muscle (the Arrector pili), which, if you're given a good scare, will cause very short hairs to stand on end.

3

2

1

John Francis and Jenny Brunt, photographed by Don Flood

Your hair (long or short, curly or straight) can be divided into three sections, and knowing what the different needs are for each part is a key to gaining control of your hair.

Section 1 is the root area. This part normally needs support, although there are times when softness is needed.

Section 2 is the middle of the hair shaft between the root and end. It may need more or less support depending on the style or texture desired.

Section 3 is the ends. This is typically an area that needs flexibility, although certain looks require extra rigidity.

A good basic understanding of these three sections and their connection with support/flexibility will also help make it easier to take control and *change* your hairstyles and textures. Also remember that when you are using products they can be placed precisely where needed and can even be layered atop one another to create different levels of texture, style, and definition.

Here's another simple three-level way to look at your hair and assess what measures may need to be taken (by either adding or subtracting) in order to achieve a desired style or texture.

If there is a secret to styling success, it's in knowing the natural texture of your hair—rough, fine, coarse, smooth, etc.—and determining how much (or how little) and to what level (maximum, medium, or minimum) you will need to "enhance" it (adding products, taking away volume, etc.) in order to achieve your goal. As an example: If you have fine, limp hair you may need to "roughen" it for up styles or you may need to create lift (either at the roots or through to the ends of the hair shaft) to create styles that need varying degrees of volume.

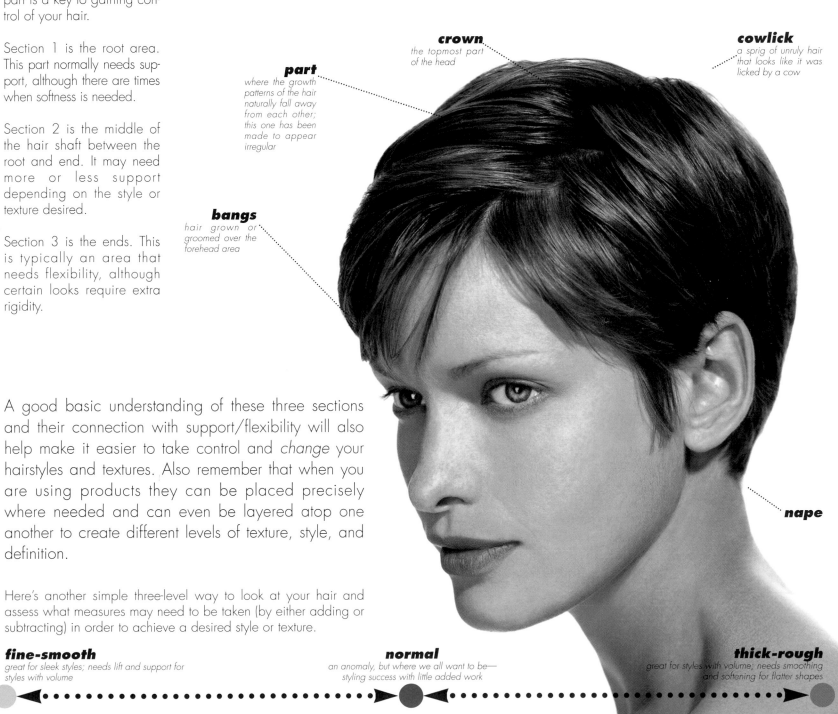

crown
the topmost part of the head

cowlick
a sprig of unruly hair that looks like it was licked by a cow

part
where the growth patterns of the hair naturally fall away from each other; this one has been made to appear irregular

bangs
hair grown or groomed over the forehead area

nape

fine-smooth
great for sleek styles; needs lift and support for styles with volume

normal
an anomaly, but where we all want to be— styling success with little added work

thick-rough
great for styles with volume; needs smoothing and softening for flatter shapes

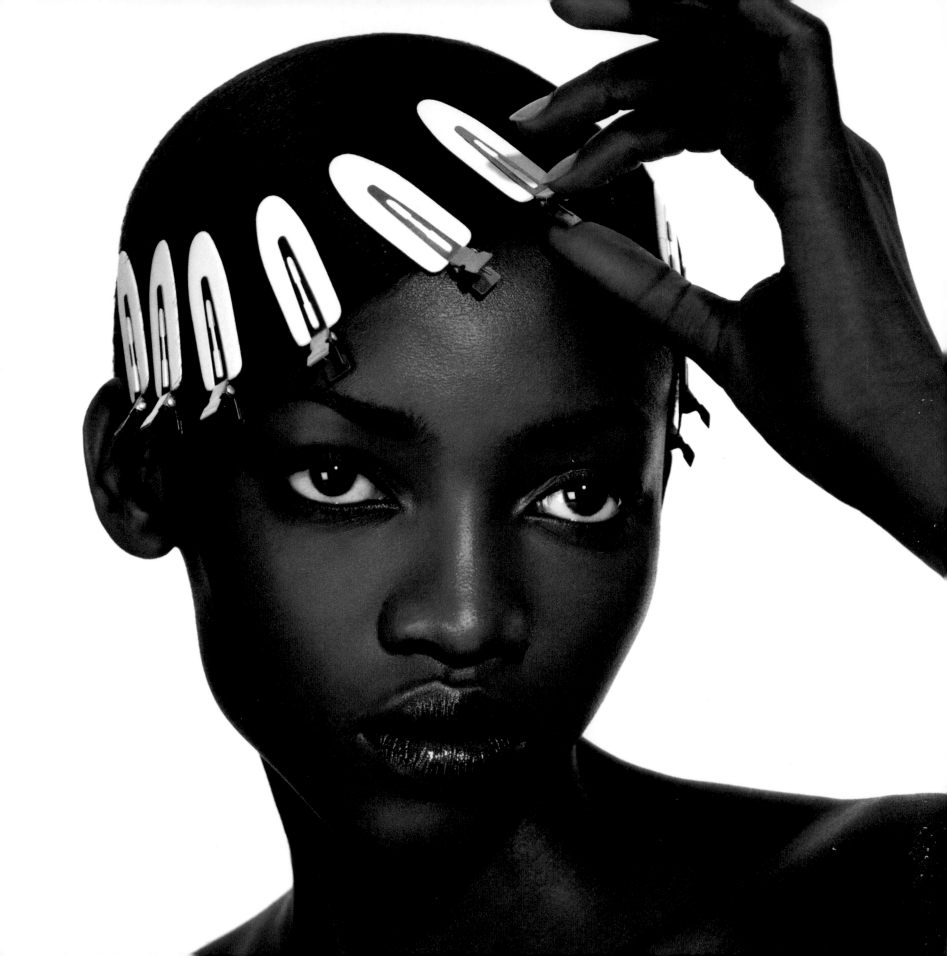

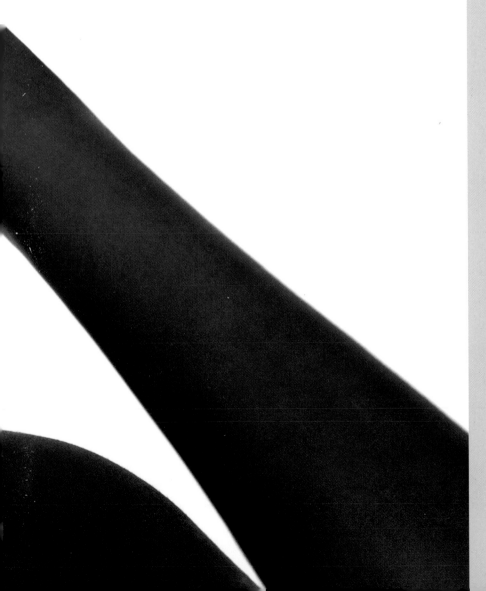

Another "secret" to having beautiful hair is using the right tools. But how do you know which ones to choose? The first and most important thing to do is determine what your hair is like naturally, then decide where you plan on taking it. If you have stick-straight hair and want lots of cascading curls, be prepared to invest in the right curlers and curling irons. This doesn't mean you're going to have to spend a lot of money to get what you want (although there are quite a few implements with hefty price tags), but you must be willing to "pay for what you get." Don't sacrifice the end result in the name of economy. However, be equally leery of laying out too much cash when it might not be necessary. The next few pages will give you some direction.

do-dads

~ After straightening Oluchi's hair, I placed a number of styling clips along the front hairline to keep it in place while she had her makeup done. These particular clips are specially made with plastic shields to prevent denting of the hair. If you want to see if they worked, turn to page 139 and check it out.

Oluchi, photographed by Don Flood

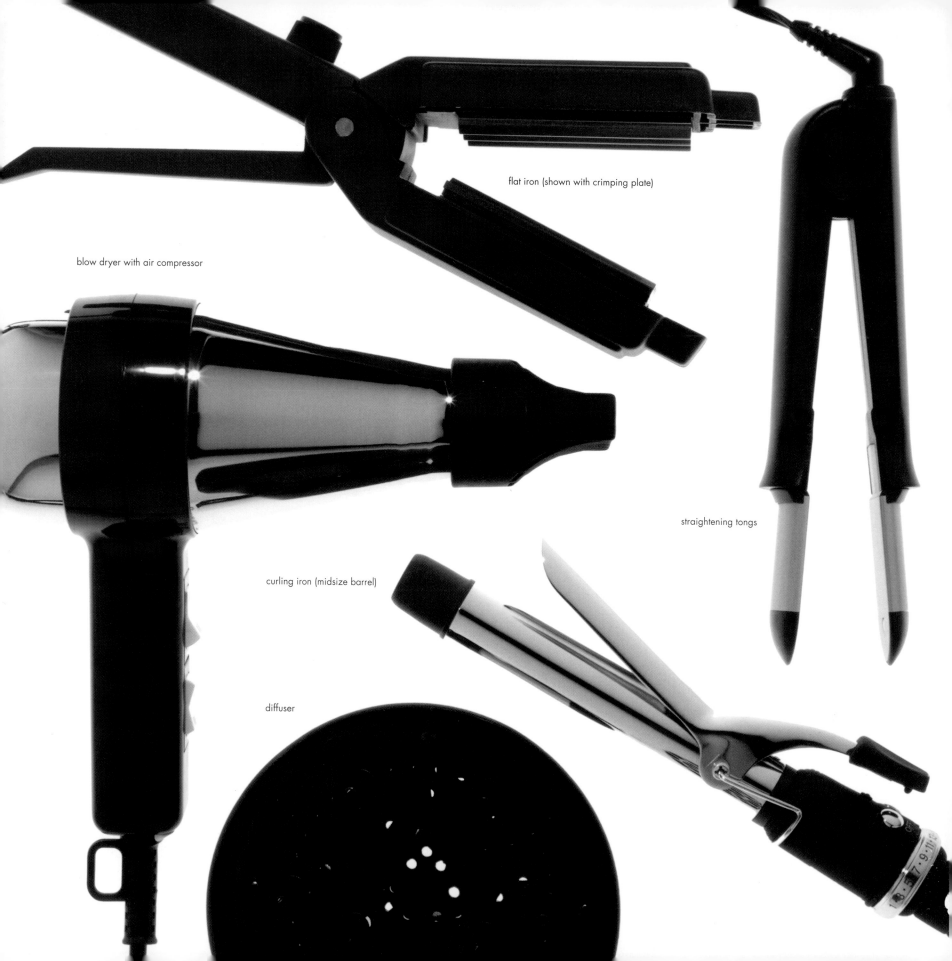

flat iron (shown with crimping plate)

blow dryer with air compressor

straightening tongs

curling iron (midsize barrel)

diffuser

A lot of the tools shown here (and on the next few pages) are categorized as "for professional use only," meaning that they can be somewhat difficult for the consumer to use (or even find). However, I think it's worth your knowing what these things are, because a good stylist may be using them on your head. Besides, if you love to work with your own hair, you may want to consider owning or at least trying them out for yourself.

power tools

blow dryers—

Choose a dryer that has balanced weight in your hand. It should also fit comfortably and not be too heavy. Be sure that it has protective screens over the fan mechanism in back (to prevent hair from getting sucked in). Choose one with a long power cord (for mobility). A blow dryer should also have at least 1,200 watts of power. Personally, I prefer somewhere around 2,000 watts—more power speeds up drying and styling. **However, when using a dryer, be careful not to overdry your hair**. It should come with an air compressor (the piece that looks like a vacuum cleaner part that everyone throws out; you need it) and have three heat settings (low, medium, high), along with one for cool air. (Even though many consumer-use models may not have all four settings, there are some models available with built-in heat sensors. These automatically cool themselves down to prevent overdrying.)

curling irons—

These hot little devils have barrels (the metal cylinder you wrap your hair around) that come in a variety of sizes, from slim as a pencil to the diameter of a can of hair spray. Obviously, look for one that is appropriate for your styling needs. It should also have more than one heat setting, fit easily in your hand, and have a clamp that is easy to open and close.

flat irons—

These are for straightening, crimping, and waving hair. If you're the type that likes to style your hair a lot, look for one that has detachable plates (like the ones pictured here). It, too, should have more than one heat setting.

straightening tongs—

Smaller and slightly more compact than a regular flat iron, these are good for straightening short hair and bangs, and detangling. A word of caution: All irons used to take quite a long time to heat up; now it takes no time at all. Regardless, never leave one on unless you plan to use it; it could melt down your whole vanity. And for heaven's sake, always watch what end you're grabbing for! Note: Keep the plates and barrels of any ironing implement clean. Styling products build up quickly and make these tools extremely hard to use, not to mention unsanitary. I spray and wipe them down with oven cleaner at least once every few days.

diffuser—

This optional attachment is for "softening" the airflow from a blow dryer, making it great for drying naturally curly hair (so as not to lose the curl) and heating up hair that's been set in rollers.

screen clean The screens on the back of dryers easily accumulate dust and hair. The blockage of airflow can cause the dryer to burn out. If your screens are not detachable for regular cleaning, periodically wipe them down with a damp cloth.

all still lifes in "Do-dads" photographed by Jay Zukerkorn

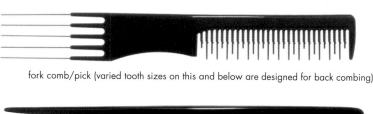

fork comb/pick (varied tooth sizes on this and below are designed for back combing)

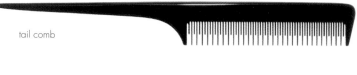

tail comb

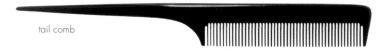

tail comb

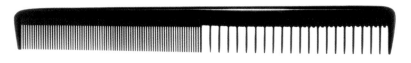

fine- to medium-tooth comb

fine- to medium-tooth comb (both of these are best on shorter hair)

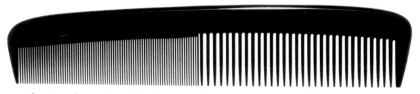

fine- to medium-tooth comb (for longer hair; bigger size is easier to handle)

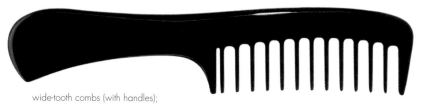

wide-tooth combs (with handles);

the one below is great for combing products through hair

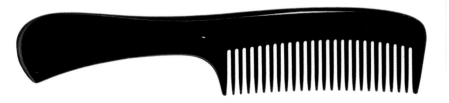

combs

fine- to medium-tooth combs—

A stylist's favorite for use while cutting hair, blowing it out, back combing, detangling, etc. However, any comb that you use in blowing out your hair should be made of hard rubber, since plastic can melt under the extreme heat of a dryer.

wide-tooth combs—

Best for combing conditioners through the hair and for blowing out textures from kinky to curly. Finer-tooth versions can be used *after* the hair has been initially straightened to get out even smaller kinks. (I use these combs to begin straightening kinky and curly hair, because they are easier to manage than finer-tooth combs, which can easily get caught in the hair.)

tail combs—

Best for sectioning hair while blowing it out and getting it out of the way (using a styling clip) when applying anything from conditioners to chemical processes.

fork combs and picks—

For "opening up" or separating curls or kinky hair. I prefer using hard rubber and plastic ones, which I find gentle on the hair. However, specifically for lifting and styling, I'll use a plastic version with a metal fork end. (The metal is even finer than plastic and makes it easier to lift a wave with more precision, leaving the overall finished look undisturbed.)

comb alone Not all combs are created equal; they come machine- or handmade, and there can be a quality difference between the two. The best comb to buy is seamless (a seam is made by the meeting of two halves of a mold). Often a machine-made comb will have excess bits of plastic hanging off of a few teeth, and these can catch, pull, and even cut your hair.

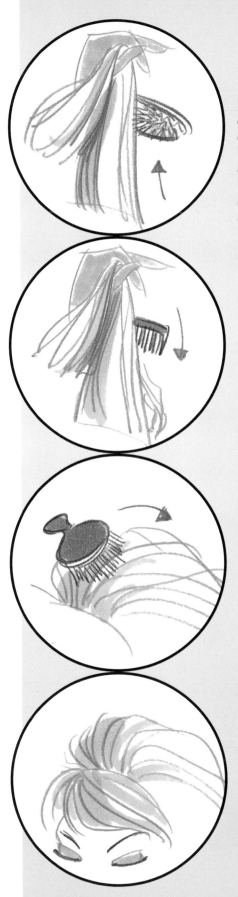

just teasing

In the old days, it used to be called "teasing." However, "back combing" is the accurate term, because it describes what you do—comb the hair from the back. Simple as it is, it's an amazingly effective technique and is used in many photo images.

1 Take a manageable section of hair in hand, using a tail comb. Comb (or brush) the section smooth.

2 From behind, back comb to create a base; start low on the hair for less support and density. **Support and density increase the higher up the hair shaft you go. Determine what amount you need using the three-level method from page 31.** It's best to use a comb for more manageability, although a brush is good for very large areas. The more the hair is texturized at the start, the better the results. Try adding a spritz of holding spray.

3 Take a brush and lightly smooth out the hairs in front to camouflage the back combing. (You can use a comb for this, but it is likely to be much harder.)

Keep in mind that you can back comb just in spots. For instance, lightly in the front for added lift, or at the crown for height. Take a look at pages 89 and 109 for examples where back combing was incorporated as part of the styling process.

parting company

You know those great zigzaggy parts that look like they just happen naturally? Well, there is an easy trick to making them that takes just a little practice.

Using the pointy end of a tail comb, quickly squiggle (or swivel, as the case may be) through the hair area you want parted. The actual "trick" is keeping the tip of the comb at an angle and in constant contact with your scalp as you run the comb along.

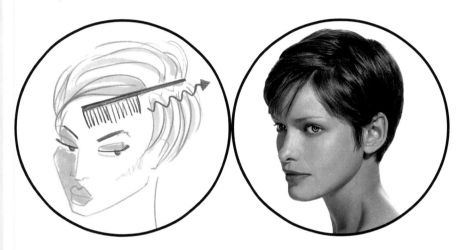

Here's another quick trick: Once you've sectioned your hair and want it out of the way, you can use a tail comb to keep the hair in place instead of a styling clip. Just twist the sectioned hair against the scalp and fasten with the "tail" end of the comb, the same way you've seen people use a chopstick or a pencil.

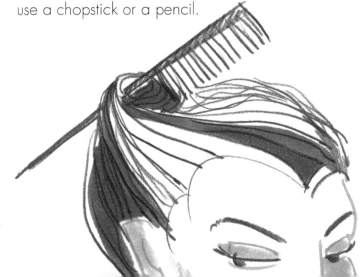

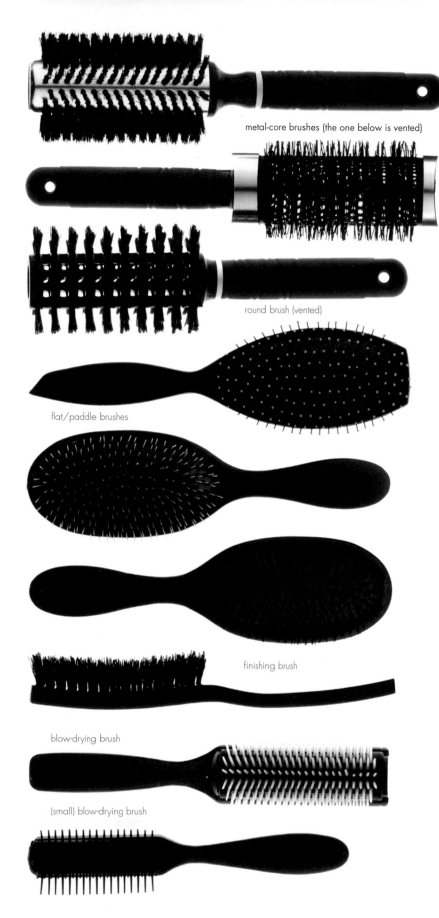

metal-core brushes (the one below is vented)

round brush (vented)

flat/paddle brushes

finishing brush

blow-drying brush

(small) blow-drying brush

brushes

blow-drying brushes—

Typically, the first brush used when blow drying your hair into smooth styles. They come in lots of sizes, with varying amounts of bristles (personally, I prefer ones with nine rows). Smaller sizes are good for working with shorter hair and can be useful for getting into hard-to-reach places (such as behind the ears). It's a good idea to have a small and a large one.

round brushes—

Used to "polish" the hair to a fine, smooth, glossy-finished texture. Also used to create flips, bends, waves, turned-under looks, and volume. Choose one based on your own specific type of hair: For fine hair, use one with densely placed, soft bristles; the thicker the hair, the thicker (less densely placed) and harder the bristles should be. I prefer brushes with only natural bristles, because I find them to be both gentle *and* effective on the hair.

flat/paddle brushes—

Great for "brushing out" a variety of hair textures, especially long hair, first thing in the morning or during the day. A paddle brush can also be used to blow hair straight and polish *after* prestraightening with a blow-drying brush.

vented brushes—

The vents allow direct airflow from the dryer through the hair, heating it more evenly and speeding up the drying process. These brushes are great for quick styling but are not the best brushes to use for polishing or smoothing the hair.

metal-core brushes—

Designed to act as a sort of one-step blow, heat, and curl tool with the metal barrel center acting as a hot roller. This speeds up the drying and styling process and can give you an easy, loose curl if you allow the hair to cool down with the brush still in place. **Note: Frequently applying intense heat to your hair can leave it dehydrated and over-blown**.

finishing brushes—

Most commonly used by pros and made mainly with natural bristles (which I prefer) or natural in combination with nylon. Shapes vary from rectangles to ovals to squares. The main difference between these and other brushes is the density of the bristles (and quality, from soft to rigid), which allows them to be used after the initial "blow out" to comb out sets and to build and back comb hair into sculptural shapes. (Another type of finishing brush, used mainly to style wigs and hairpieces, has metal bristles. I don't recommend them for real hair unless you use one that has ball tips and bristles planted in a flexible rubber base.)

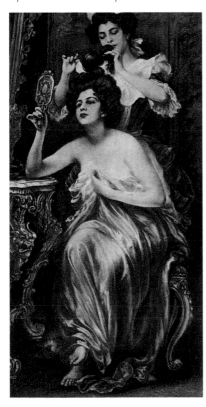

Over the centuries, the brushing of hair has taken on an almost mythical aura. It seems nothing is so alluring as a woman stroking her long, wavy tresses. But don't believe all the hype. Will brushing cause hair to grow? Not really, but stimulating the scalp is one way to loosen any build-up from around the follicles, which can clog pores. Is brushing hair (a hundred times) good for it? Yes and no. Brushing to detangle and keep hair managed is good; excessive pulling and yanking is not. Will brushing hair make it shiny? Well, sort of, if you consider that brushing helps to distribute oil secretions from the glands surrounding hair follicles. *Drawing courtesy of Corbis-Bettmann*

brush tip Hairbrushes need to be broken in; the more you use one, the softer and more conforming to your hair it will get (and the more effective it will be).

A clean tool will be more effective and last longer. Brush the teeth of a comb with a brush, and comb **brush off** the bristles of a brush with a comb to loosen and remove hair. Then, if you like, you can wash them with detergent or even shampoo and quick dry them with a dryer.

getting the brush Natural or man-made bristles? Natural bristles have softer tips and, overall, tend to be finer, more flexible, and break in easier. (Incidentally, you can buy one made with either boar's hair or hardened silk bristles.) Man-made bristles are usually less expensive and grip the hair well, but are often rigid and inflexible. Combo brushes (real and nylon bristles) are a great alternative.

How do you know if you have a good brush? I test them with something I call the "grip and **brush rush** glide" method. Simply, a good brush is a brush that grabs hold of the hair but allows for an easy brush through to the ends. Any good brush should do this.

neutral ground Sometimes for a lot of styles it's necessary to "neutralize the direction" the hair grows. As an example, in order to get absolutely symmetrical bangs you may need to neutralize a cowlick, otherwise the hair will stick up in that spot. Other times the direction your hair grows may be toward the back, but the look requires the hair to go forward. The easiest way I've found to alter this situation is to take my dryer and a blow-drying brush in hand and, while concentrating heat at the root area, brush the hair back and forth until it hangs straight. Then, once I'm sure I have neutralized it, I apply a stream of cool air to keep it that way.

"Polishing" is a term used to describe the action of **polishing** smoothing hair and giving it a nice, natural shine. This technique involves using hot air from your dryer first, quickly followed by cool air to seal the cuticle layer, in unison with constant twirling motion and slight tension from your (round) brush for the best results. (Just heating, cooling, or brushing alone won't do it.)

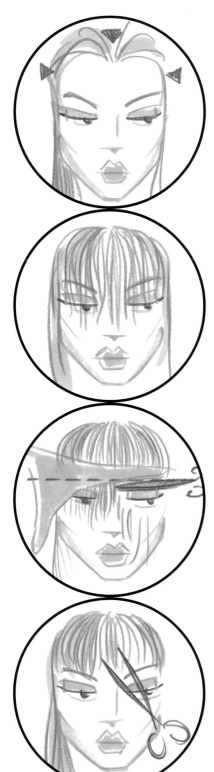

bangs a lot

Cutting bangs is difficult but not impossible. It just takes patience to get them perfect. (And it doesn't help knowing one wrong move can screw them up.) If you want to try it yourself, here are a few simple guidelines.

1 Bangs typically start about an inch back from the front hairline and above the temples. Comb bangs forward and straight down against the forehead. Determine the line and level in advance of cutting. If you have a cowlick, this is the time to neutralize it.

2 With the middle and pointer fingers of one hand, "scissor" a smallish section of hair and hold it in place, allowing the portion to be cut to hang *below* your fingers. Then take the shears, and with one blade resting against the underside of your clasped fingertips, snip atraight across.

3 Before cutting each successive section of hair, a bit of the previously cut section should show, serving as a guide for more accuracy.

4 If the finished line is not as precise as you'd like, the best alternative is not to try cutting again. (You could end up clipping them away to nothing.) However, a way to camouflage mistakes can be accomplished by taking the shears and lightly notching at the bang line, creating an irregular, more natural-looking edge.

Tip: For the casual look, you can forgo accuracy and twist all the bang hairs together, pull them lightly down the middle of the face, and snip across. Incidentally, this tip works best on straight to wavy hair with just a little body.

shears

Most people don't cut their own hair, leaving that to a stylist. However, a lot of us will trim the edges now and then. Here is a simple overview of the basic cutting tools.

standard shears—
Smooth bladed for general cutting and shaping of the hair. Also for notching the edges of hair (by eye) to give it a more natural look. Best for cutting straight lines. I prefer the three-finger-rest version for control and comfort. The swivel version is for cutting at angles *up* into the hair. (Better shears also usually have small plastic or rubber bumpers on the handles, acting as shock absorbers.)

thinning and notching shears—
Great for removing bulk from hair, making it easier to style. Thinning softens the edges of a blunt cut. (Be careful when thinning curly or kinky hair, as the clipped pieces tend to contract inward, creating a hairy undergrowth.) Notching shears are a specialized version of thinning shears, to create even more irregular edges and layering.

razors—
For cutting softly sculptural, nonprecision shapes. Also used to remove short hairs from around the neck area. (An open pair of sharp shears can do the same.) This is also the type of razor used by barbers for shaving.

clippers—
More a man's barbering tool, but they are often used to trim and shape hairlines and eyebrows, and manicure the edges of short haircuts.

the cutting edge Avoid dropping a pair of shears (at any cost). Any chink along the blade will render them dangerously ineffective.

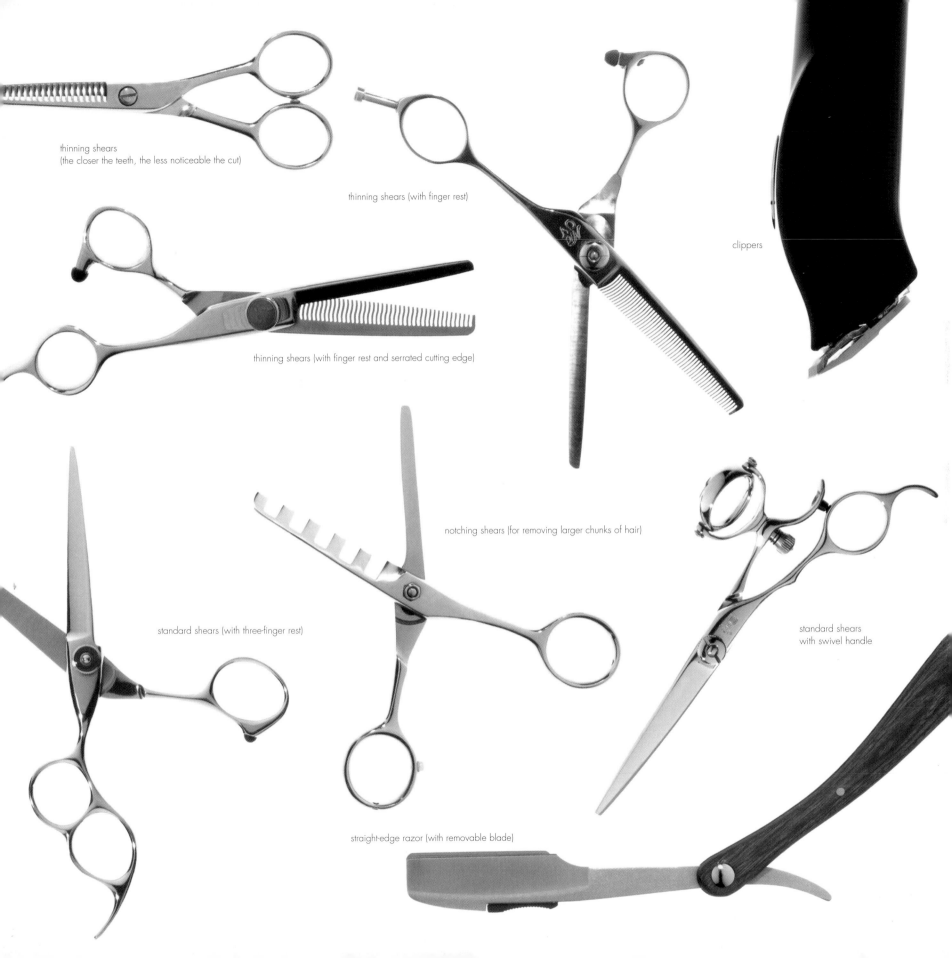

thinning shears
(the closer the teeth, the less noticeable the cut)

thinning shears (with finger rest)

clippers

thinning shears (with finger rest and serrated cutting edge)

notching shears (for removing larger chunks of hair)

standard shears (with three-finger rest)

standard shears
with swivel handle

straight-edge razor (with removable blade)

clips and pins

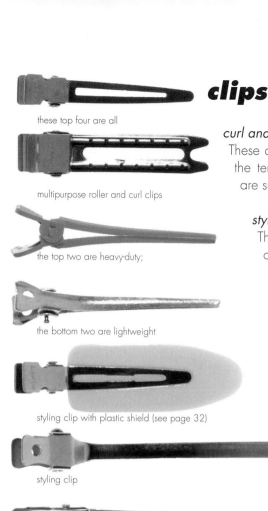

these top four are all

multipurpose roller and curl clips

the top two are heavy-duty;

the bottom two are lightweight

styling clip with plastic shield (see page 32)

styling clip

styling clip with ventilation holes

holding clip

wave clip

holding clip

curl and roller clips—
These clips have a space toward the back by the tension spring for the roller's edge. They are suitable for any type of roller.

styling and holding clips—
These are designed specifically to hold areas or pieces of hair in place (or out of the way) while you work on overall definition, direction, and wave. Some have plastic shields to prevent denting of the hair.

wave clips—
These clips are designed to catch the ridge of your wave and hold it in place until it dries. The key to using them successfully is to never place them on the hair if it is too wet, or too deeply (squeezing in too much hair), as doing either will leave jagged dents in your waves.

bobby pins—
These "pins" are usually flat with plastic ball tips. However, some have small ridges along the top side to allow for the variations in the thickness of your hair. They are used to hold styles in place, or for pinning up more creative looks. Also great for affixing ornaments and flowers to the hair.

hairpins—
These U-shaped objects come in a variety of sizes (and weights), from the almost invisible to heavy as a coat hanger. The invisible ones are used for detailing up hairstyles and to hold very fine hair in place. The heavier the pin, the thicker and the more hair you can keep in place. They are also useful for holding ornaments, flowers, and hats in place (with or without the additional use of bobby pins).

these top three hairpins were all used on the up-twist style on Rachel, to the right

extra strong and long bobby pin

this is a great pin
for holding ornaments and flowers in the hair

this pin has a hooked end to keep it secure

assorted small and lightweight hair and…

bobby pins

this one was used to secure
the ponytail on page 45

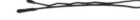

this hairpin was used to secure
Elizabeth Hurley's hair, invisibly, on page 14

to the right: Rachel Shane, photographed by Nicolai Grosell

the up-twist

Doin' the twist. Brush your hair back, as though you were ready to make a midposition ponytail (see page 45). Grasping all of it in one hand, twist and turn the hair up (either to the left or right) and fasten with a long, strong bobby pin (coming in from the opposite side).

Add one long bobby pin up through the bottom of the hair (close to the scalp) to further fasten it, make it sturdier, and keep it in place.

Continue twisting the hair and folding it into itself (adding pins if necessary), working your way up to a spiky (or loose) "spray" at the top. If you started twisting too low at the beginning, you won't have enough hair at the top for effect. If you started too high, you'll have too much.

Work the "spray" by hand, in irregular sections, as though you were arranging flowers. Use a little hairspray, if necessary, to keep pieces in place. A little below shoulder-length hair will give you the best results.

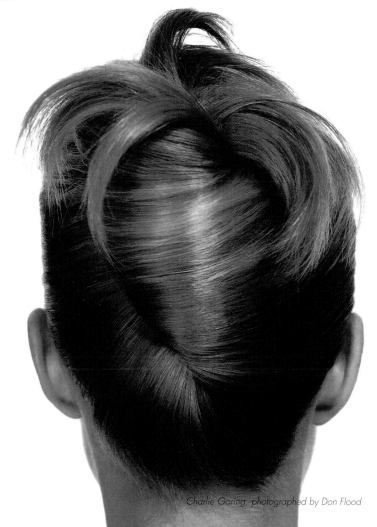

quick change This was the second hairstyle done on actress Rachel Shane the day of her shoot. The first is the "hip" texture seen on page 109. To create this style, a reverse version of the up-twist, I brushed her hair out and back, added a bit of clay groom, and gathered it into a ponytail. But instead of pinning the hair up, I fastened it down. The sprigs around the front were made by pulling out and lightly spraying random sections of hair.

Charlie Goring, photographed by Don Flood

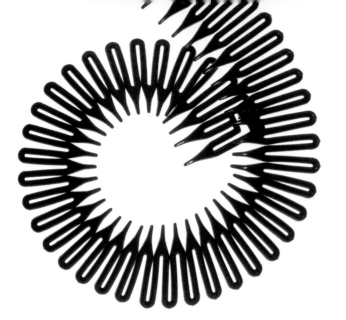

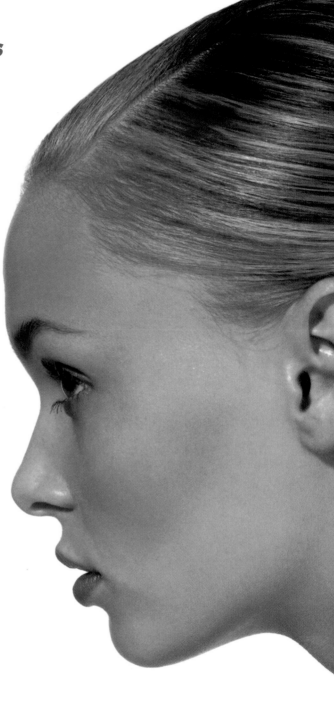

coils and elastics

comb coil—
An alternative to a headband, for pulling back the hair. Look for small ones that practically disappear into the hair.

elastics—
Used mainly for ponytails, falls, and special hair effects.

Fabric covering prevents hair breakage and snagging.

These elastics, with hooks on both ends, look like miniature bungee cords and are great for holding the hair in place. You wind them around and hook the ends together, attaching the hair exactly where you want. One drawback: Although they are readily available in Europe, they are hard to find in the States.

Tiny elastics (even ones used for dental braces) are great for creating little hair sprigs and other special effects.

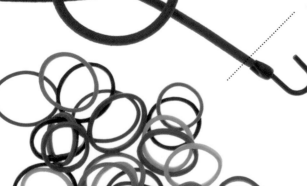

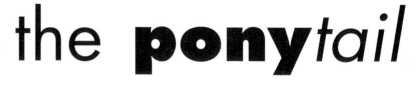

the **pony**tail

Melissa Brown, photographed by Don Flood

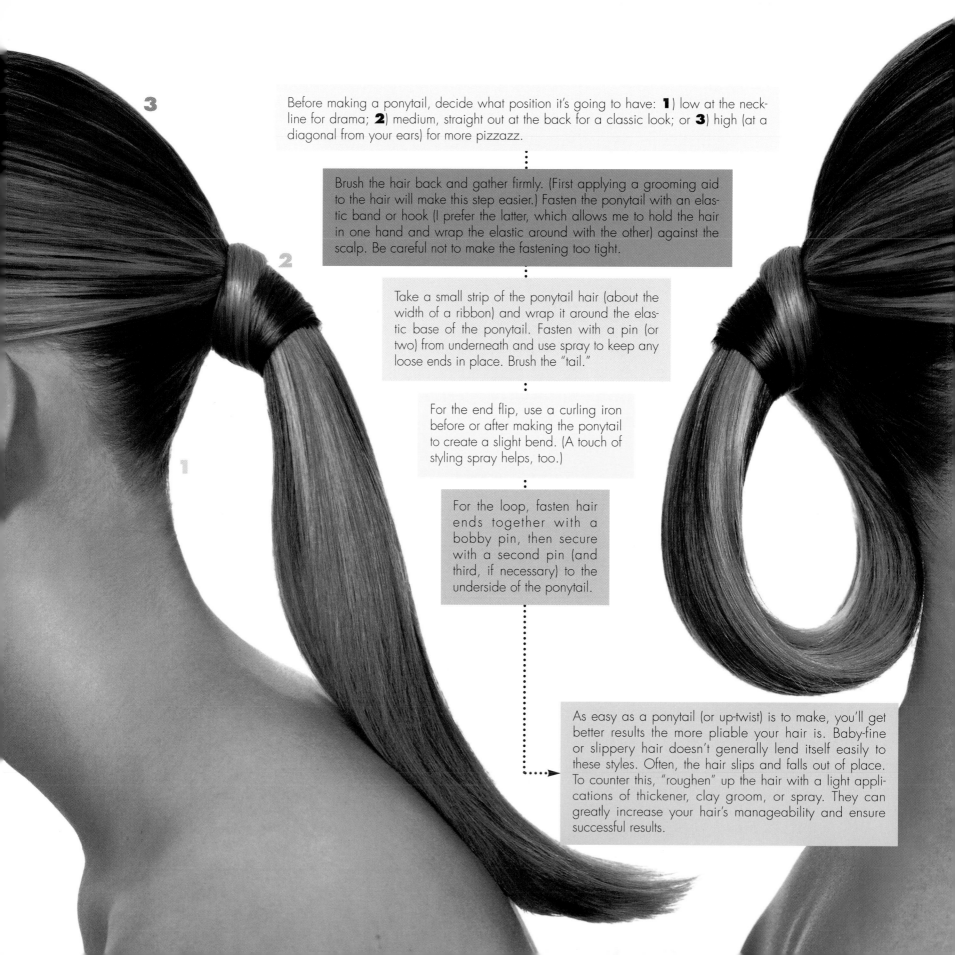

Before making a ponytail, decide what position it's going to have: **1**) low at the neckline for drama; **2**) medium, straight out at the back for a classic look; or **3**) high (at a diagonal from your ears) for more pizzazz.

Brush the hair back and gather firmly. (First applying a grooming aid to the hair will make this step easier.) Fasten the ponytail with an elastic band or hook (I prefer the latter, which allows me to hold the hair in one hand and wrap the elastic around with the other) against the scalp. Be careful not to make the fastening too tight.

Take a small strip of the ponytail hair (about the width of a ribbon) and wrap it around the elastic base of the ponytail. Fasten with a pin (or two) from underneath and use spray to keep any loose ends in place. Brush the "tail."

For the end flip, use a curling iron before or after making the ponytail to create a slight bend. (A touch of styling spray helps, too.)

For the loop, fasten hair ends together with a bobby pin, then secure with a second pin (and third, if necessary) to the underside of the ponytail.

As easy as a ponytail (or up-twist) is to make, you'll get better results the more pliable your hair is. Baby-fine or slippery hair doesn't generally lend itself easily to these styles. Often, the hair slips and falls out of place. To counter this, "roughen" up the hair with a light applications of thickener, clay groom, or spray. They can greatly increase your hair's manageability and ensure successful results.

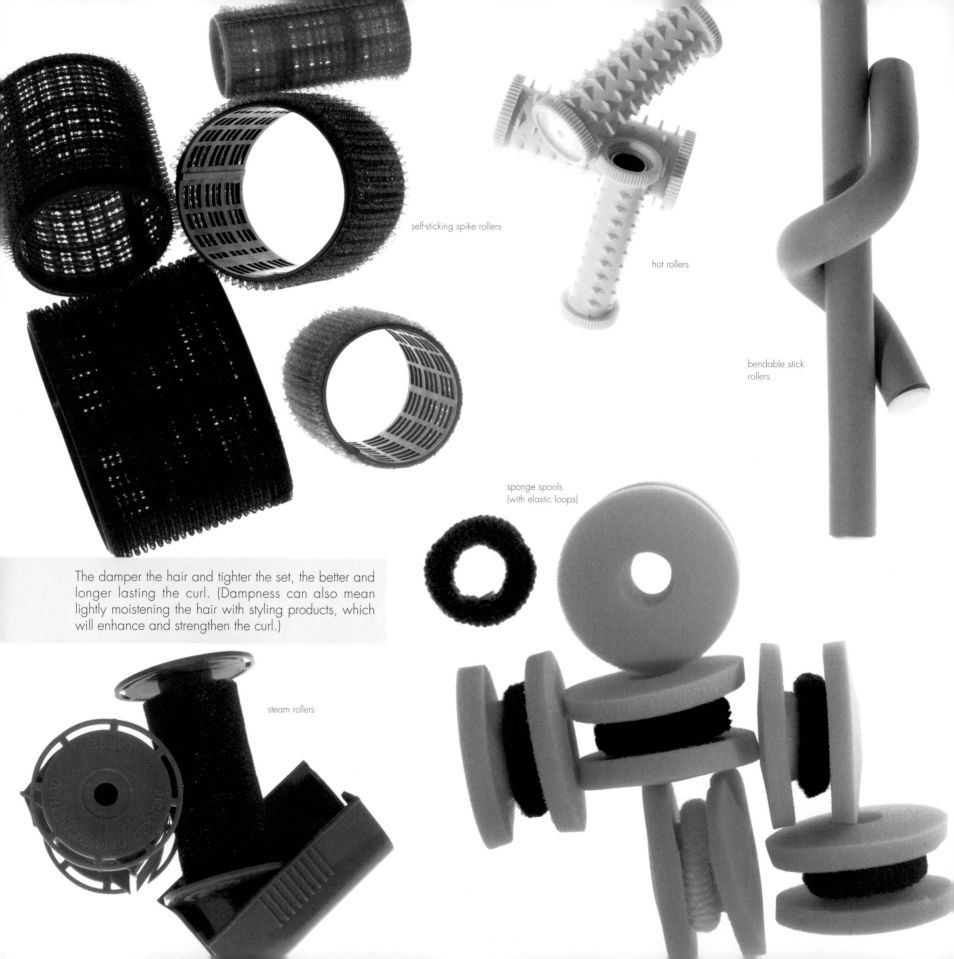

self-sticking spike rollers

hot rollers

bendable stick rollers

sponge spools (with elastic loops)

The damper the hair and tighter the set, the better and longer lasting the curl. (Dampness can also mean lightly moistening the hair with styling products, which will enhance and strengthen the curl.)

steam rollers

rollers

hot rollers—

These rollers come with their own self-heating case and work by using dry heat on the hair, allowing the strands to reconfigure into a curl or wave, or giving hair extra body. Good for straight to wavy hair.

steam rollers—

For use on dry hair only, steam rollers have a vented core wrapped in sponge, which allows for steam to penetrate the hair shaft. This prevents dehydration of the hair and in many cases can give you a stronger set than hot rollers. However, steam rollers may not be suitable for those with hair that reacts adversely to moisture, activating more curl and frizz, and compromising the desired texture and style.

self-sticking spike rollers—

The spikes on these rollers hold the hair in place during rolling and setting. The rollers have ventilation holes for easy drying and come in a wide variety of sizes. One drawback: They can easily snag hair, especially the type prone to tangling. If you run into this problem, try pretreating the hair with a silicone product.

sponge spools—

For making spiral curls (by twisting damp hair first, then rolling), these are extremely gentle on the hair. Porous sponge also soaks up excess moisture. (The elastic loop is for keeping the hair in place.) However, don't expect to get a great curl if you have straight, dry hair, as these will not give you enough support. Best for hair that has some curl in it already.

bendable stick rollers—

Like an art tool for curling your hair. Wind the hair around and lock it in place by bending the stick. More fun than practical, but they can create some interesting shapes.

roll with it

For a basic set using self-sticking rollers:

1 First, decide the direction(s) the curls or waves should take. Then, make a determination as to the amount of curl or wave you want.

2 Take a section of hair and brush it into a peak. (Make the sections the same width as the rollers.) Apply styling spray or creme groom to each section to enhance the curl and make it more manageable. (Whether you're setting your hair damp or dry, adding styling products will ensure better results.)

3 Use the roller to comb hair into place, going as close to the ends as possible. Twist the extended part around and tuck it under rolled hair using your fingertip. (Going all the way to the ends is more difficult to manage.) For longer hair, self-sticking rollers may need to be held in place with clips.

4 Lightly apply styling spray to rolled hair at the roots for lift and over entire set to smooth flyaway hairs.

5 Apply diffused hot airflow (using a diffuser and dryer or a cap). When the hair is completely dry, allow it to cool.

6 Unwind the rollers carefully, and brush the hair into place according to the desired style.

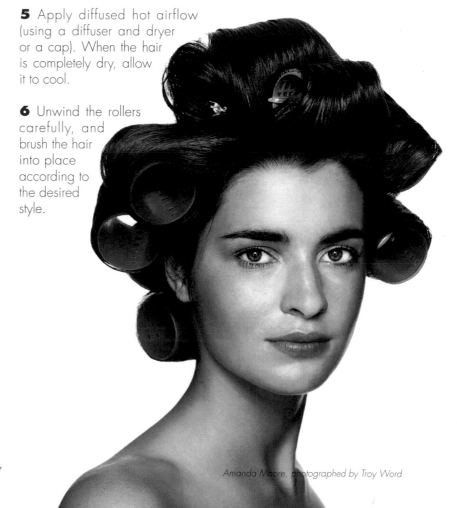

Amanda Moore, photographed by Troy Word

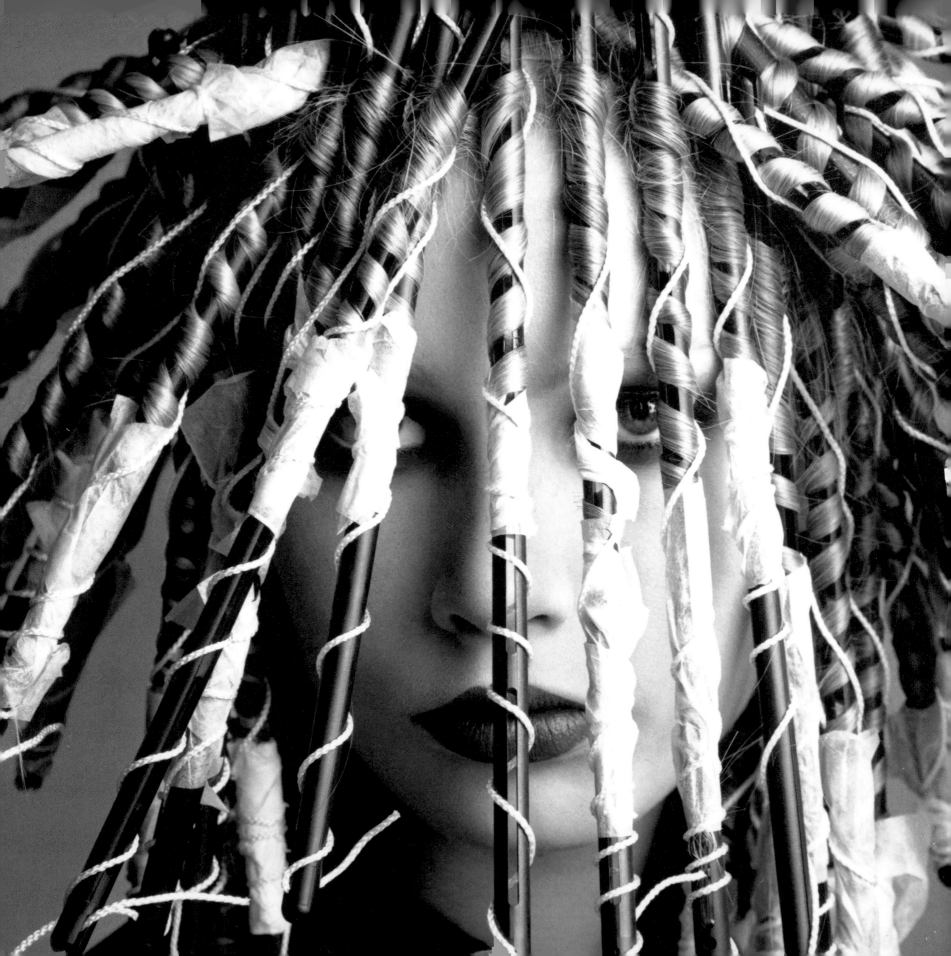

Do you ever wonder what it would be like to wake up some morning looking completely different from the way you did the night before? With little more than a bottle and a brush, a dark vamp can be turned into a blond bombshell. Miss Straight as an Arrow can be transformed into Lady Godiva with a perm set that will last her well beyond just one night of fun. And, amazingly, each of us has the ability to make these changes ourself. Whereas once these things were time-consuming, expensive, and in many cases dangerous, advances in chemical formulations and application techniques have brought them out of the dark ages. Today the drawbacks are few. However, remember that any time you use chemicals on something as vulnerable as your hair, it is wise to exercise a bit of caution. You might not know when too much is too much until it is too late. Happily, though, your hair should grow back unharmed, and you can try again.

medicine
mane

~ *Gorgeous Kirsty Hume had to submit to a seemingly endless five-hour prep for the photo on this page (and its "finished"-look portrait on page 51). Her hair had to be twisted, tied, and papered on more than fifty perming rods. Though the photo was done mainly for effect, the outcome is a great example of how extravagant you can get when styling and setting hair.*

"Perms" have been with us for a long time (flip back to the opening page to see how far we've come from looking like part of a GM assembly line), and today the process can be done in any number of ways, with or without heat, and with a variety of setting devices, using actual permanent or regular rollers or long sticks (seen on page 48). Which method is chosen is usually determined by the desired result, with each giving different configurations. You can create spirals and tight or loose curls, add waves, crimp, or even perm over existing curls to open them up, making them larger and looser. It's also a great way to give normally limp, fine hair some much-needed texturizing to make styling easier. However, a "permanent" wave (or curl) treatment will only affect the hair it

permanents

comes in contact with; any that grows out afterward will be unaffected. Furthermore, since a certain amount of natural relaxation and oxidation will occur, extra upkeep is necessary to maintain a perm's effect on your hair at the highest level.

Permanents as a body or root lift. A root perm, so named because it is performed at the root of your hair, is helpful if you want to a) create a stronger curl or wave pattern in an area where the hair is flat as a result of being too fine or limp (or because it is weighed down by length), or b) create a style that requires more initial lift or width. A body perm can add overall shape to your hair and can be done as subtly as a simple bend in the hair

or a soft wave pattern (which will add support for styling, especially any kind of curling and roller sets, and natural drying). And don't forget, perming is also an effective way to add volume to your hair.

Spot perms as a great "temporary" permanent solution. A spot perm can be used to help touch up specific areas, like the front hairline, where you may need to create height for a particular style, or match up textures where one area is inconsistent with another, as in a patch of straight hair next to curly or frizzy (which occurs more frequently than you might think).

~ The finished portrait of Kirsty Hume. After unwinding her hair, I used a touch of silicone to help define and separate the curls. I kept the brushing to a minimum, and then only from underneath, using a large-tooth comb, so as not to disturb the volume and shape.

perm alert As handy a styling and texturizing aid as permanents can be, there are some drawbacks, not the least of which is the smell of some of the chemicals necessary in the processing. Frequent improper treatments can damage the hair and the scalp (though developments in the field have helped many of us avoid any mishaps). And you should refrain from multiple chemical processes, meaning anything more than two at one time (for instance, going from black hair to blond is already a two stepper), because they can easily result in disaster, which I have seen many times. And even though the thought may be tempting (especially from an economic standpoint), don't perform a perm at home on your own unless you really know what you're doing.

Kirsty Hume, photographed by Patrick Demarchelier for Harper's Bazaar

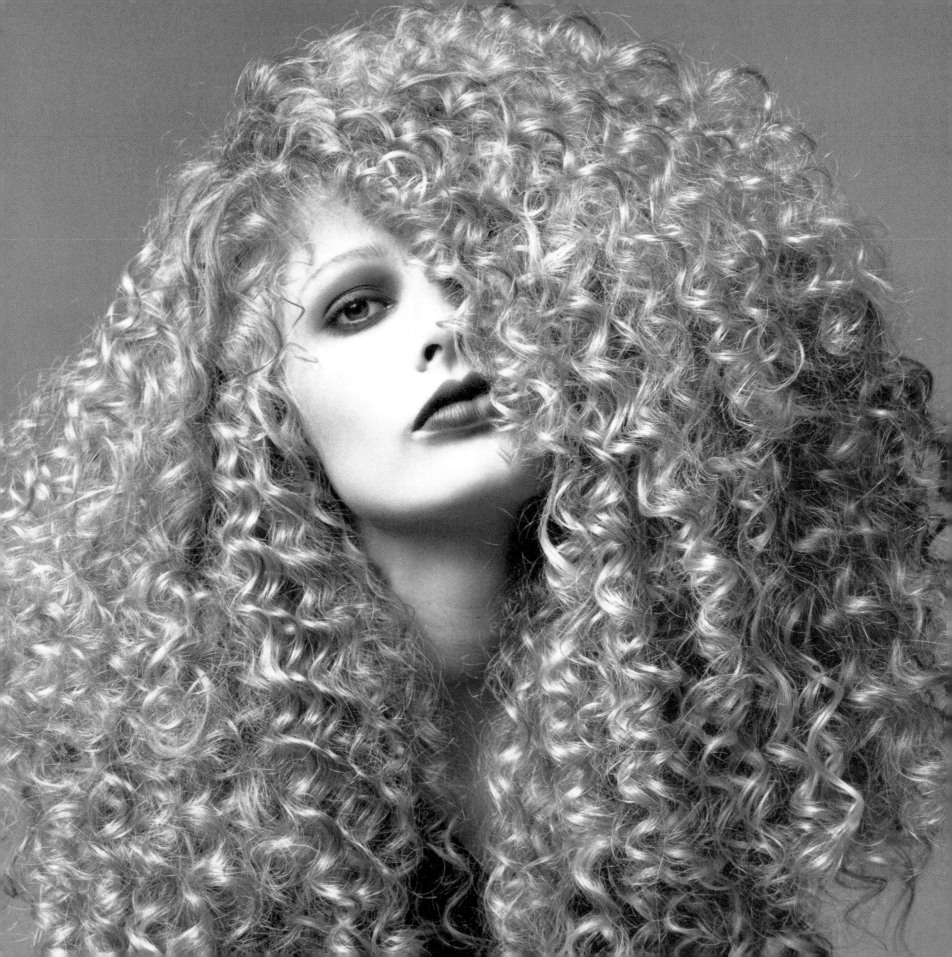

From my childhood I recall the "only your hairdresser knows for sure" line from hair color advertising. The fact that my mom colored her own hair only reinforced the mystique around coloring. I also remember other women in my neighborhood, many of them my mother's friends, swearing that their hair was *naturally* copper or platinum (and on some unfortunate occasions orange). Well, hair color has come a long way. It is no longer a shameful secret. In fact, today's hair coloring formulas can leave your hair looking and feeling even better than it did when you started out. This is an added benefit to some great improvements in the color formulas themselves, not to mention that clients today love to boast about having their hair colored by the best salon special-

coloring

ists, at several hundred dollars a head. So if you haven't already done so, why not give it a try? You may find yourself hooked.

fine find I'm an advocate of hair color for many reasons, not the least of which is the flexibility it gives to hair that beforehand was limited in its options. Fine, limp hair, especially, can benefit from the process. Hair color expands the cuticle layer, making it more texturized, which in turn allows for more manageability. You can also control the level of volume and texture you add to your hair by varying the amount of highlighting or coloring. As a rule of thumb, any small amount of coloring will add some rigidity and support. As you increase the level of application, volume and texture follow in tandem. Your once unworkable hair now responds to your styling manipulations and isn't slipping out of your hands.

color product basics

temporary hair color

Should last only a few weeks, more or less, depending on how stringently and often you shampoo. "Stains" the hair topically, and only the surface of the hair strands is involved. These products work best on porous hair (which attracts more pigment) and lighter-colored hair. (The darker your hair color, the less apparent the results). Be aware that some temporary formulas can be especially messy to work with, and the color is so "cosmetic" it can rub off on clothes, and even be removed in one shampoo.

semipermanent without peroxide

Also a staining process, but more long lasting than temporary (up to six weeks). Again, starting with porous or light-colored hair will give you the best results. Previously processed hair may color so well that you'll want to choose a shade lighter than you anticipated (example: medium brown to achieve dark brown).

semipermanent with peroxide

Formulated with a low-volume peroxide to open up the cuticle layer—just enough to allow pigment into hair previously resistant to coloring. However, it can cause oxidation of the natural color, lightening it slightly. So depending on color choice, darker roots can show with time.

permanent

Complete hair color change until your roots grow in. Uses peroxide (and ammonia) to open the cuticle layer; hair is not only "permanently" colored, but effectively texturized, which is great for hair that is normally hard to manage. However, color oxidation can occur, especially on golds and reds, which will appear faded over time and need color fresheners.

~ *Model Heather Dillon is undergoing the most basic of color treatments: a temporary hair color. Here it was intended only to intensify and refresh her natural shade. Look for a beautiful before shot of her on page 26, and an amazing after (with some straightening) on page 54.*

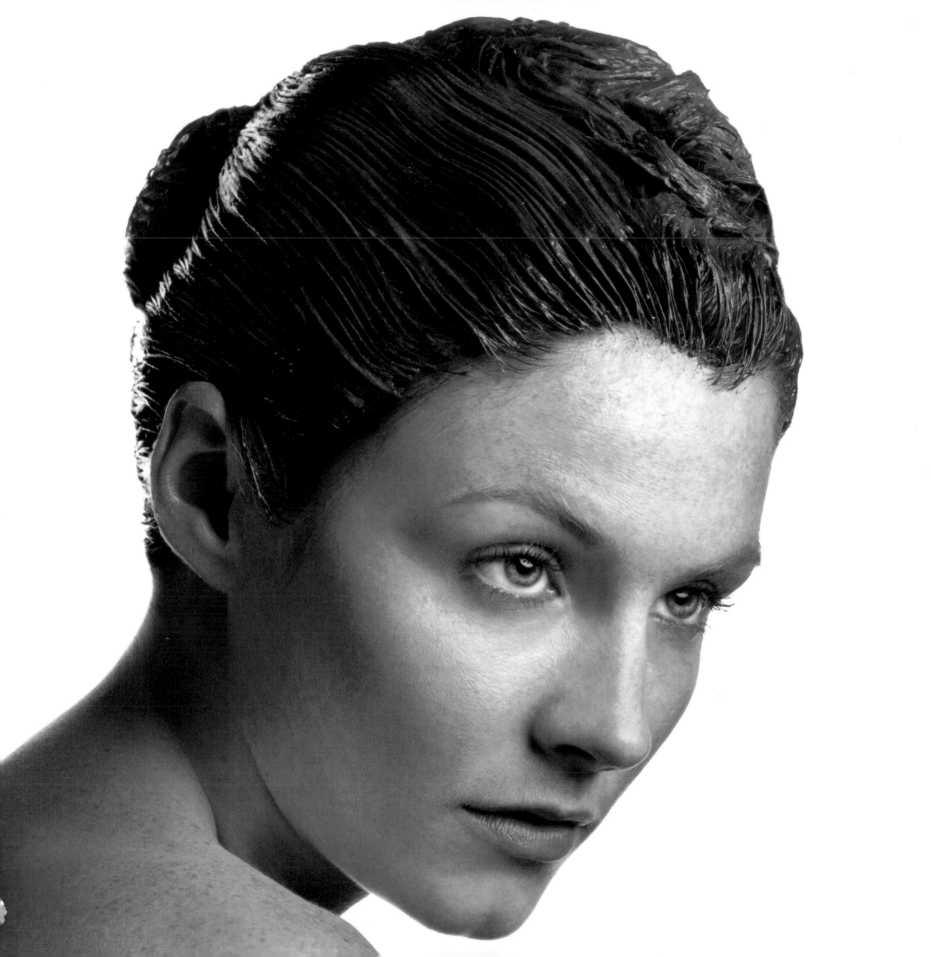

color notes

The colors we see are a reflection of light, period, and your hair is no exception. If you won't take my word for it, turn out the light and see how everything goes gray. Another consideration is how colors affect each other. Remember the color wheel from school days, with the colors divided among primary and secondary ones? By mixing some we'd get purple or orange (and if we mixed too many, we'd end up with something the color of mud). Coloring your hair follows the same principles with one major exception: your hair's natural pigment is either red or brown based or a mix of the two.

You need to answer a few basic questions before you start: What color do you want and will you be able to achieve that successfully? How long do you want it to last? How much of a change do you want? What amount of maintenance are you willing to commit to?

Whatever you come up with, if this is your first time, I recommend that you take the safest route and go to a colorist. His or her advice will prove invaluable to you in the long run. If you decide to take matters into your own hands, literally, I suggest opting for the simplest course (especially if you are new to this). Those choices include a temporary color rinse or enhancer. These treatments are more or less foolproof, and the experience will prepare you for the big stuff down the line.

tint hint
Tinted conditioners are a great way of "freshening" up your hair color. (However, if you are blond [natural or processed] be aware of possible color change and staining.)

never say dye
I use the word *color* instead of *dye*. That's because the term *dye* is old-fashioned. Besides, the connotation is one of absolute permanence and seriousness. *Color* (and *coloring*) has a more positive sound, and when it comes right down to it, it is precisely what you're doing.

at-home basics
Always read the manufacturer's instructions. That's what they're there for, and you may come across things you hadn't considered. *Try a strand test.* Very important if you are not sure of the color and how it may affect your hair. *Try a patch test.* If you have sensitive or allergy-prone skin. *Applying color.* Most kits come with applicator bottles and gloves. However, using a brush to apply color is much more accurate. Why not investigate owning one yourself? *When in doubt.* If you aren't sure and you think you need help, you can always speak to an experienced colorist by calling the 800 number on the box.

~ *Here is Heather after her hair was color enhanced and straightened. What an amazing change, considering that both looks, before and after, are equally beautiful options.*

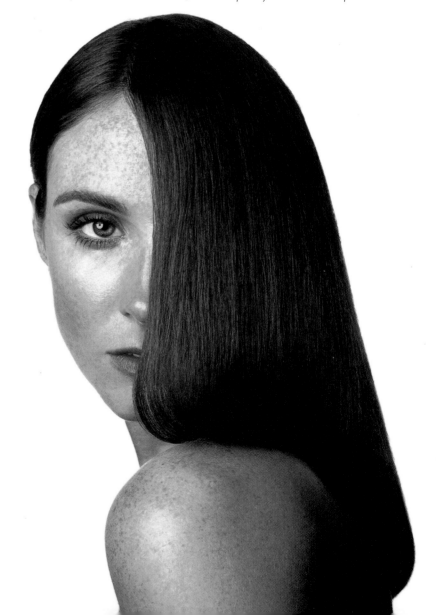

54

blondie

Do blonds have more fun? Maybe not in everything, but certainly when it comes to hair coloring, they have a distinct advantage. Especially if you have very light-toned blond hair, your options are practicallly limitless. However, just the opposite is true, too. Blond hair (especially if it is color processed) is very susceptible to staining and color change. It is wise to avoid any hair products with tint or coloring.

redhead

If you're a redhead, you'll find the most pleasing results if you opt for warm shades of brown and auburn when coloring your hair. If you have light red hair, you should also be able to go to a strawberry blond quite easily with a one-step process utilizing a "high-lifting" tint. However, if your ambition is to go blond, beware of ending up with orange, especially if you are attempting this at home. Best to leave it to a pro.

brownie points

Always remember when coloring brown hair that the natural pigment usually has red or gold undertones. Keep this in mind especially when attempting to lighten it, as it can go brassy. Darkening it is not a problem, but avoid coloring so deeply that all natural highlights are taken out.

gray matter

Since gray hair is a mix of dark with light hairs, it's tricky to process in one way. The term "covering over" refers to someone who just wants to hide spots or pieces of gray, but is not looking to strip all the rest of the hair of pigment in order to address these few strays. Another option is to highlight or lowlight the hair in places to lessen the appearance of gray.

black out

Two things to be aware of: First, some black pigment is so strong you'll have to strip the color first (sometimes many times) and then add one back in. This is a double process; never underestimate how it can affect your hair. Second, coloring over black (with black) can sometimes take out natural highlights, making your hair look one-dimensional.

A word or two about henna. The big allure with this product is that it is natural, therefore environmentally friendly to work with. However, when working with any natural substance, it can be harder to control the results. And henna can conflict with some chemical processes. (If you are planning one, discuss it with your colorist first.) Nevertheless, it will give you pretty good coloring, especially if you start with lighter-shaded hair and are looking to go just a bit darker, and it is well known for giving hair plenty of shine.

trio of Jenny Brunt, photographed by Nicolai Grosell

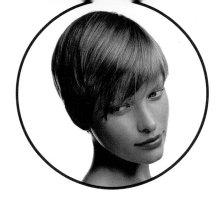

Highlights add brightness to the hair, lowlights add depth. There are basically two ways to highlight/lowlight your hair. One is done by separating and coloring many individual hairs all over the head. The second gives a chunkier look, and is done by coloring the hair in sections.

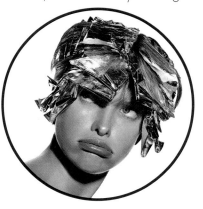

Foils are the best way to get a precise placement of color for highlighting/lowlighting because you can isolate individual hairs. Also the foils act as little incubators to speed up the coloring process. However, you can highlight/lowlight your hair with a treatment called *baliage*. This is a more abstract method that uses the edge of a comb, dipped in coloring then run over the surface of the hair. This technique can look spotty if not done well. Look for a specialist.

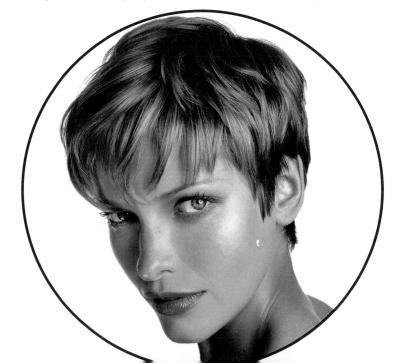

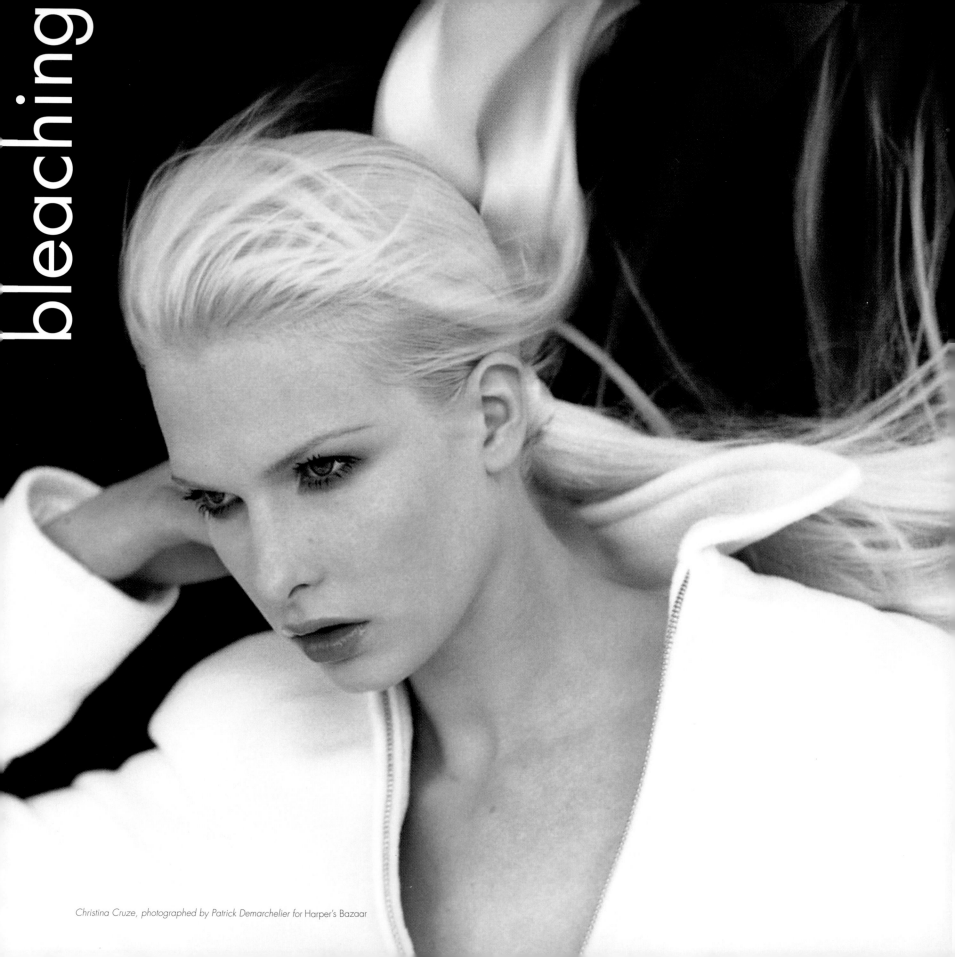

bleaching

Christina Cruze, photographed by Patrick Demarchelier for Harper's Bazaar

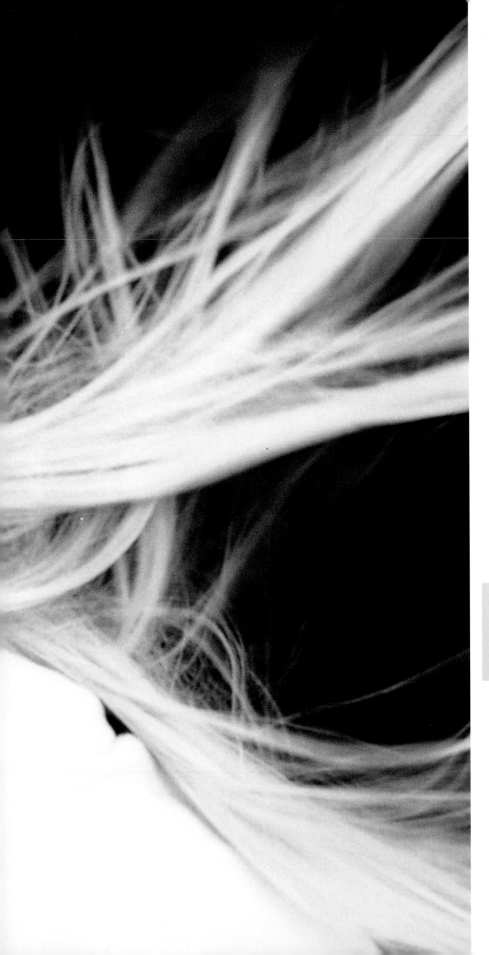

Though the practice is very common, you should never underestimate the process of bleaching your hair. Basically, what you are doing is stripping the hair of all pigment (using different levels of peroxide), leaving it virtually translucent. (Check it out when it's wet; your hair looks like fishing nylon.) And sometimes this process has to be done over and over in one sitting to be successful. (The active ingredient in peroxide stops working after it has dried.) Then you need to add color back in. You never want to leave bleached hair absolutely colorless—it will look unfinished. Even when you are finished, your hair is still very vulnerable and will need to be maintained with the utmost care, including touch-ups to the roots, conditioning, and the like.

As serious as some of this may sound, there is a definite upside. Double processing your hair (bleaching first, then coloring) makes it amazing to style. In fact, the texture can hold almost any shape you give it. This is the very reason it was so easy for Marilyn Monroe to get those fabulous upswept hairdos all through the fifties. If you need more recent proof, check out Ashley Judd's glamorous portrait on page 141.

what you see
Is not always what you'll get. Often the color of hair in a commercial is heightened for effect. The extra vibrancy of a particular shade (like a bright auburn red) is necessary for it to show up properly on film. It's unlikely that you'd need or want it to be that intense on your own head.

Once double processes were developed in the twenties, Hollywood was quick to capitalize on the look. On film, certain types of very light blond processed hair, especially, appeared to glow and shimmer like pale silver, giving rise to the term *platinum blond*. Incidentally, the most famous of them all, Jean Harlow, actually started out with very nondescript sandy blond hair. *Photo courtesy of Kobal*

hollywood blond

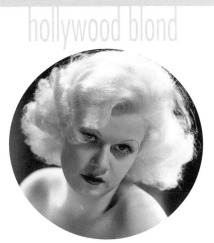

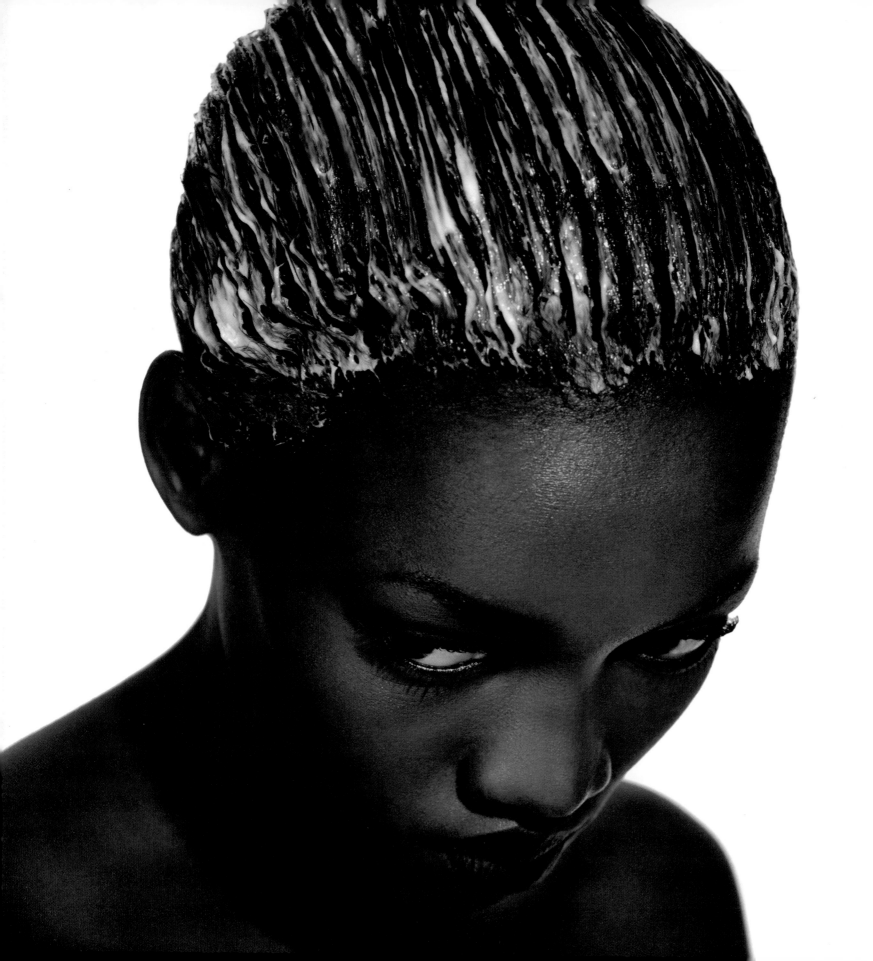

Relaxers are among the strongest chemical processes that you can use on your hair, second only to bleaching with a high-volume peroxide, and should be used only under the best circumstances. Personally, I suggest that you get a professional chemical technician to do it for you. Your colorist might do, but be sure to check to see if he really knows what he is doing before committing to this (or any other process, for that matter), because you have to live with the results, good or bad. If you feel comfortable enough doing it yourself at home, just make sure you have the manufacturer's 800 number readily available in case you run into any problems or feel uncertain about any of the directions. (Most manufacturers supply this on the side of every box. Avoid buying a product that doesn't have one.)

Basically, hair straighteners and relaxers are the same thing (with relaxing the more common term). They come in lye and no-lye formulas (although no-lye is just a milder, less effective form of lye). The active chemical ingredient in lye is sodium hydroxide, which breaks down the cuticle layer of hair, allowing it to lie flat. The longer you keep the product on, the better it works (how strong the formula must be is determined by the thickness of your hair), but again, the longer you keep it on, the more susceptible your hair is going to be to damage. It is best not to use relaxers on highlighted or permanently colored hair, and definitely not on hair that has been bleached, as this will severely weaken the hair, to the point of breaking.

For women with very curly or kinky hair who cannot satisfactorily straighten it by normal styling means, relaxing is the only option that can give them any flexibility. If done right, relaxing can make unmanageable hair manageable and less likely to break (because combs go through straightened hair more easily than curly or kinky hair). However, relaxing your hair does tend to dry it out, so you should deep condition it to keep it soft and hydrated. Otherwise it will be left unnecessarily brittle.

relaxing

Some of the best things about working with hair today are the many options available for us (stylists and clients alike) to change the things that we don't like, add what we don't have, and cover over what we don't want to see. I am referring to artificial hair, which is not meant to imply that this type of hair is not real. To the contrary, much of it is made from the real stuff. (In fact, some of the best pieces are made from human hair, specifically grown for these purposes.) There are add-ons, which include clip-on bangs and falls; wigs, which range from the full, pull-over-the-scalp creations that come in a zillion different choices to wiglets (often nothing more than a handful of extra curls sewn together); and finally, there are extensions and weaves.

hair today,
gone tomorrow

Keep in mind that wigs are not just for people who are losing their hair or have something to hide. You'd be quite surprised at how many people (and that includes the biggest superstars and models) are wearing them just for the fun of it!

wigs

A wig is fantastic if you want to change your whole look in an instant. Just be sure to choose one that fits the head properly and match it as closely as possible to your real hair color (unless the idea is to go for something completely different, in which case you'll have to make sure to

got to be real

Natural versus synthetic hair? Since hair is basically already dead, buying a wig made from a stranger's hair should be no big deal (believe me, the person who grew the hair won't miss it): it's also easy to restyle and pretty much handles like your own hair would. A couple of considerations: Expect to pay high prices for high-quality pieces, and be sure to find out what chemical processes have already been done to it in case you want to do something to it yourself, like coloring or perming (because the hair will already be weakened). Synthetic hair is pre-shaped, easy to clean, extremely resilient, and relatively inexpensive. Drawback: It doesn't always look real (although there are some fantastic fakes available) and you can't restyle it without great effort. The decision is yours.

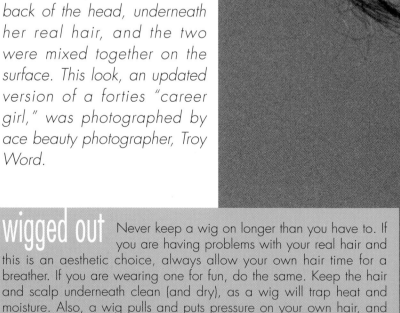

~ A large curly hairpiece was used to create this look of gravity-defying volume and curl on adorable Janine Giddings's short, fine brown hair. Starting from behind the ears (at the lower part of the crown) the add-on was clipped in place across the back of the head, underneath her real hair, and the two were mixed together on the surface. This look, an updated version of a forties "career girl," was photographed by ace beauty photographer, Troy Word.

wigged out

Never keep a wig on longer than you have to. If you are having problems with your real hair and this is an aesthetic choice, always allow your own hair time for a breather. If you are wearing one for fun, do the same. Keep the hair and scalp underneath clean (and dry), as a wig will trap heat and moisture. Also, a wig pulls and puts pressure on your own hair, and that stress can show (and be felt) over time.

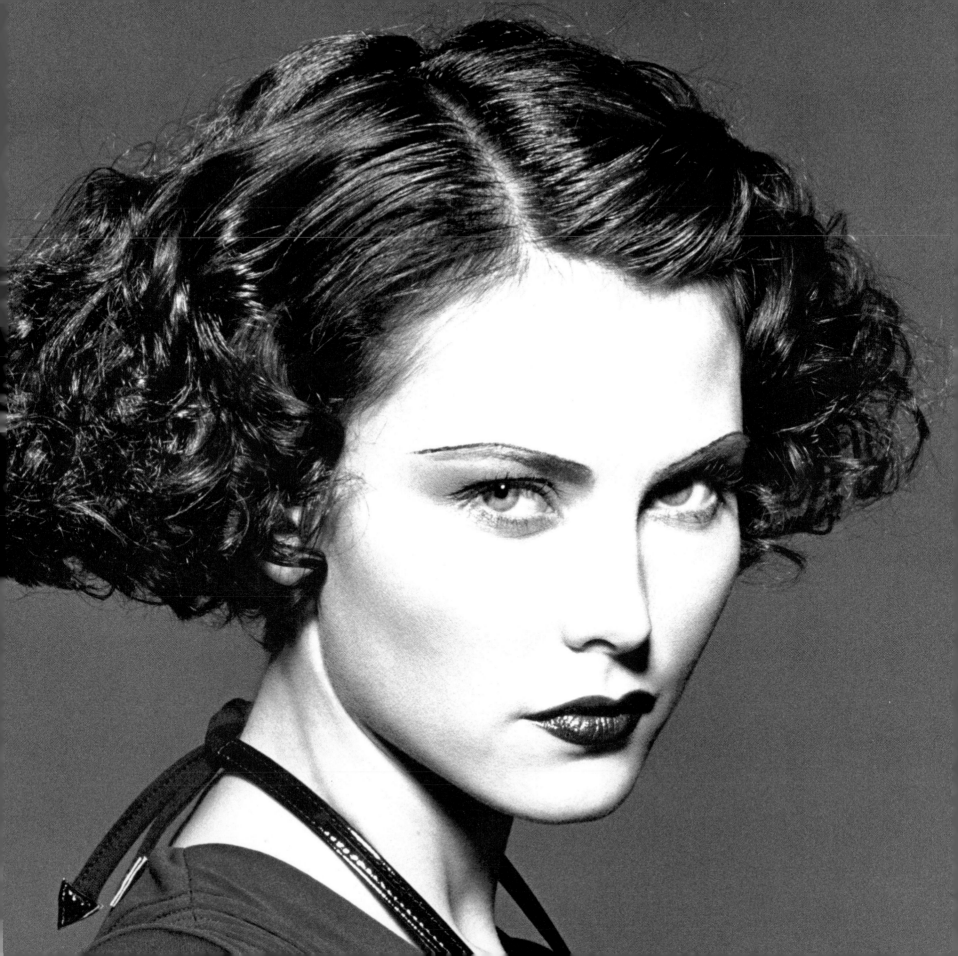

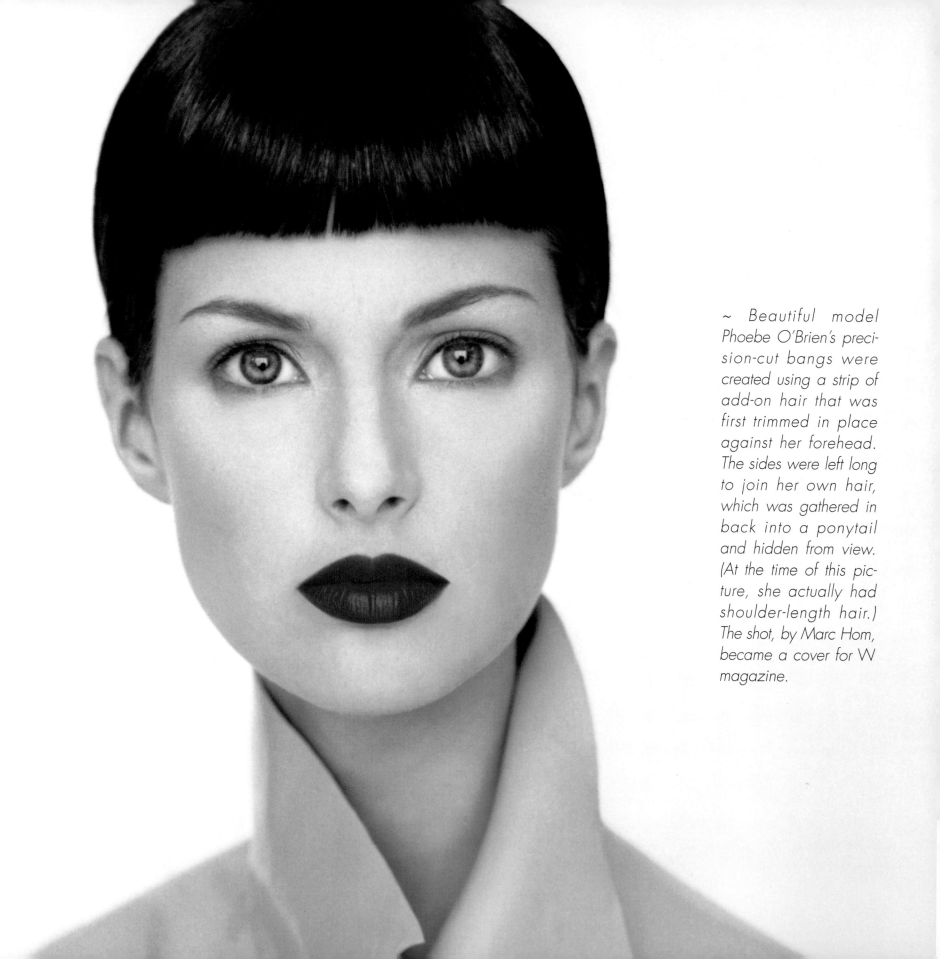

~ Beautiful model Phoebe O'Brien's precision-cut bangs were created using a strip of add-on hair that was first trimmed in place against her forehead. The sides were left long to join her own hair, which was gathered in back into a ponytail and hidden from view. (At the time of this picture, she actually had shoulder-length hair.) The shot, by Marc Hom, became a cover for W magazine.

place it correctly on your head, lest a few hairs show and the illusion is shattered); and keep it clean and tidy just like your real hair. Note: Both real-hair and synthetic wigs should be sent to a stylist for care and conditioning, because they are both susceptible to unintentional alteration of color and style.

Now, the placement of a wig is really everything, and oftentimes the trick to carrying it off is allowing your *natural* hairline to become intermeshed with that of the fake piece (or pieces). However, if that is the case, then a match in coloration of the two (your hair and the wig) is very important. (The best and most elaborate of wigs actually re-create a natural hairline, requiring a little adhesive to stay in place and an ample application of foundation makeup to hide the seams.) Still, most wig wearers will opt for that complete over-the-scalp type that is relatively easy to carry off, so long as you check to put the front in front.

add-ons

These hairpieces include clip-on bangs (like the one pictured on Phoebe, to the left), ponytails, falls (see Janine, on page 61), and wiglets (those funny little pieces of hair that sometimes fall off at the most inopportune moments if not fastened on properly). People wear add-ons for a variety of reasons, from camouflaging thinning hair patches, to adding just the right and manageable amount of panache to a look without investing the time in waiting for one's own hair to grow out or having to style it. (Remember, it is harder for some people to curl and configure their hair than it is for others.) Here again, the secret to wearing one is to make it look like part of your natural hair. So try to match the color, unless you're going for highlighting effects; secure it in place adequately (most of them come with tiny comb attachments, but you may need some bobby pins, too); and always intertwine your real hair with the add-on to hide the evidence.

falling into place

Where and how you position an add-on hairpiece is as important as the piece itself. The spot you choose to place it will determine how easy (or difficult) it will be to make it look like part of your real hair.

1 For bangs

2 For falls and add-on hair (for fullness)

3 Along the part (one inch away)

If you can't find the right add-on piece, you can easily make one yourself. Hair can be bought in different lengths and a variety of colors. Across the top of a hairpiece, the hairs are held in place by either multiple stitches or a fabric band (the former is lighter and easier to camouflage, the latter a bit more resilient but harder to hide). Select what you need and gather it together. (You may need to tuck in and hand stitch the side edges.) Then sew your own clips into place (the best are the tiny ones used for men's toupees), and you're set. Note: Keep the pieces small and manageable at first, until you get the hang of it.

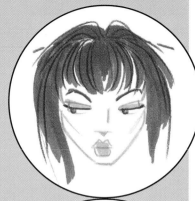

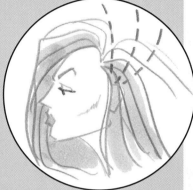

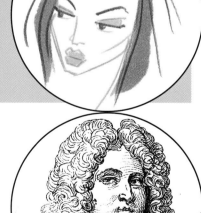

Back in the seventeenth and eighteenth centuries, men wore wigs as often as women did. In fact, the most powerful men in society wore large powdered ones (this included our own American forefathers), and the more important the individual, typically the larger and more impressive the wig. This is where the term *bigwig* comes from. *Engraving courtesy of Corbis-Bettmann*

extensions and **weaves**

First, let me make the distinction between the two, which, although some people think they are, are not the same thing. An extension is actually individual groups of hair strands that are attached to your own hair by braiding (similar to a type of knotting) to keep it in place. Extensions can be elaborate and long pieces of hair as well as shorter lengths. The wearer usually chooses them because they are relatively easy to put in and allow a great deal of freedom for styling effects. Moreover, if they are done well, extensions have a lot of movement and life. Weaves are a bit more complicated. They are actually sewn by hand, interlocking with the natural hair right up against the scalp. The real hair is first braided against the scalp, forming rows of patterned foundations that the wefts of hair are attached to. The process is time-consuming and needs upkeep (as your hair grows out, the weaves tend to loosen and will need to be tightened). But it's well worth the effort, especially for anyone who might need a breather from relaxing and straightening her hair, or any individual who finds it difficult to grow her hair to a desired length.

For someone who has never had long hair, trying either of these two methods—weaves or extensions—or for that matter putting on a wig, can be a revelation. The attraction and allure of a long mane is well known, to the point where it is an indelible part of our culture. (This goes for long hair on women *and* men.) If you have the opportunity, you should try it.

shortcut Unsure about clipping off your cherished locks? Not convinced that the latest look is right for you? Why not try on a short (or styled) wig to see if the shape suits you before you commit? Granted, a wig salon owner might not appreciate this tip, but if you are hesitant about getting your hair cut or restyled, I'd be surprised if you hadn't thought of doing it already.

~ *Basically, this is the longest wig I have ever seen. I jokingly placed it on model Leilani Bishop's head (about four inches back from the front hairline) while she was leaning against an interior studio wall. I then proceeded to brush her real hair over the top of it and continued intertwining and twisting it with her own hair as I went back, creating a very long ponytail look. Even though we were just having fun, when editor extraordinaire Polly Mellen caught sight of it, she insisted photographer Sante D'Orazio take a picture for the* Allure *story we were working on. (Just so you know, the wig ends below the hips; Leilani's own hair stops at midchest.)*

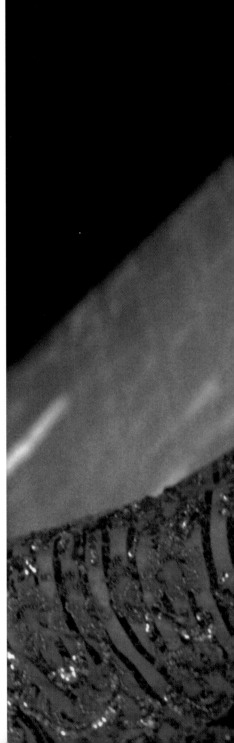

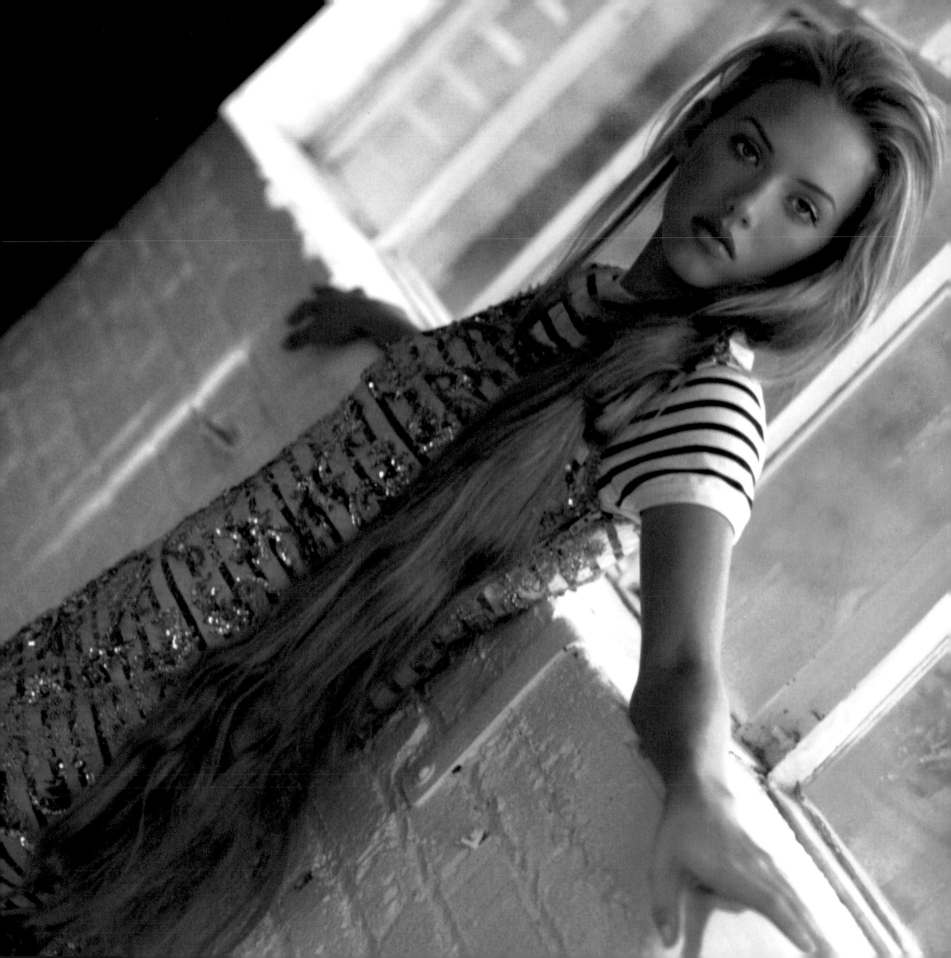

At this point, you must make a determination as to whether or not you are happy with the hairstyle and texture you have. If you are, then continue on. If not, maybe it's time for some action.

The key to accomplishing great hairstyles starts with a great cut. But the question is, How do I get one? I can't tell you exactly what to do, because I don't know you, but speaking as a stylist with many years experience, I can give you some very sound advice on what I feel the best options are for your hair.

I know that getting a haircut can sometimes be a woman's (and man's) worst nightmare. The stress may be so great for some that they schedule an appointment and

getting clipped

don't even show up. Or they do go, and their anxieties cause them to end up with something they're not happy with. Try not to let it get to you. You're thinking that's easy for me to say because I'm on the other side. But I can ease the tension with a little at-home, presalon preparation that you can do before you go. (Remember, this is supposed to be a pleasurable experience, not a tax audit!)

How do you find a good stylist? A referral is a great way to find one, but not always. Most people are very loyal to their stylists and will refer everyone and anyone to them. So to be on the safe side, ask yourself if you really like the hairstyle and texture of the person doing the referring. Also, see if she is able to manage the style with

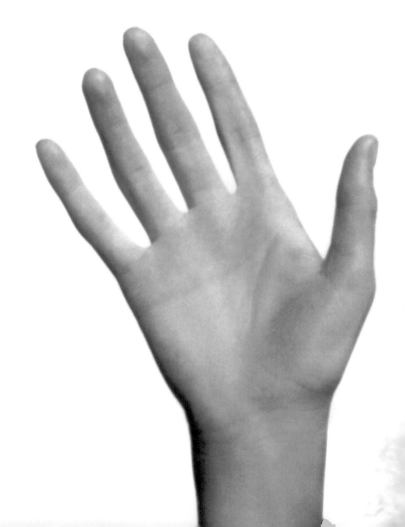

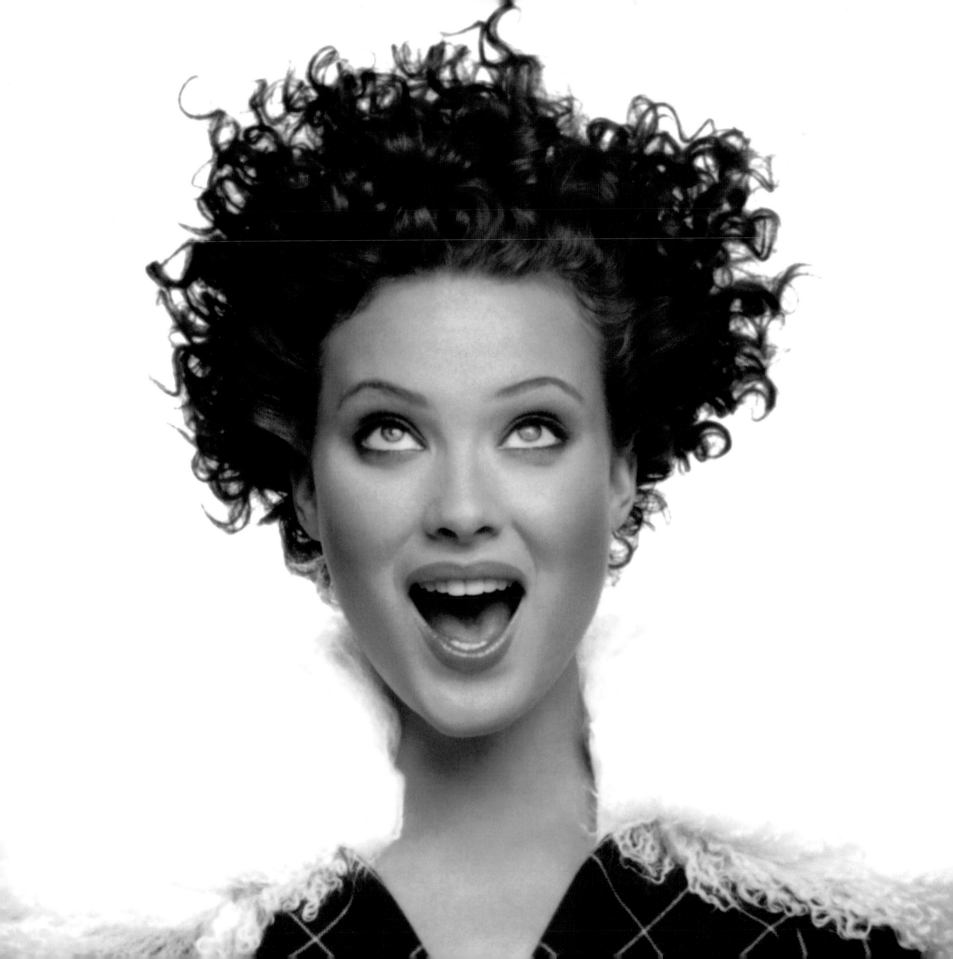

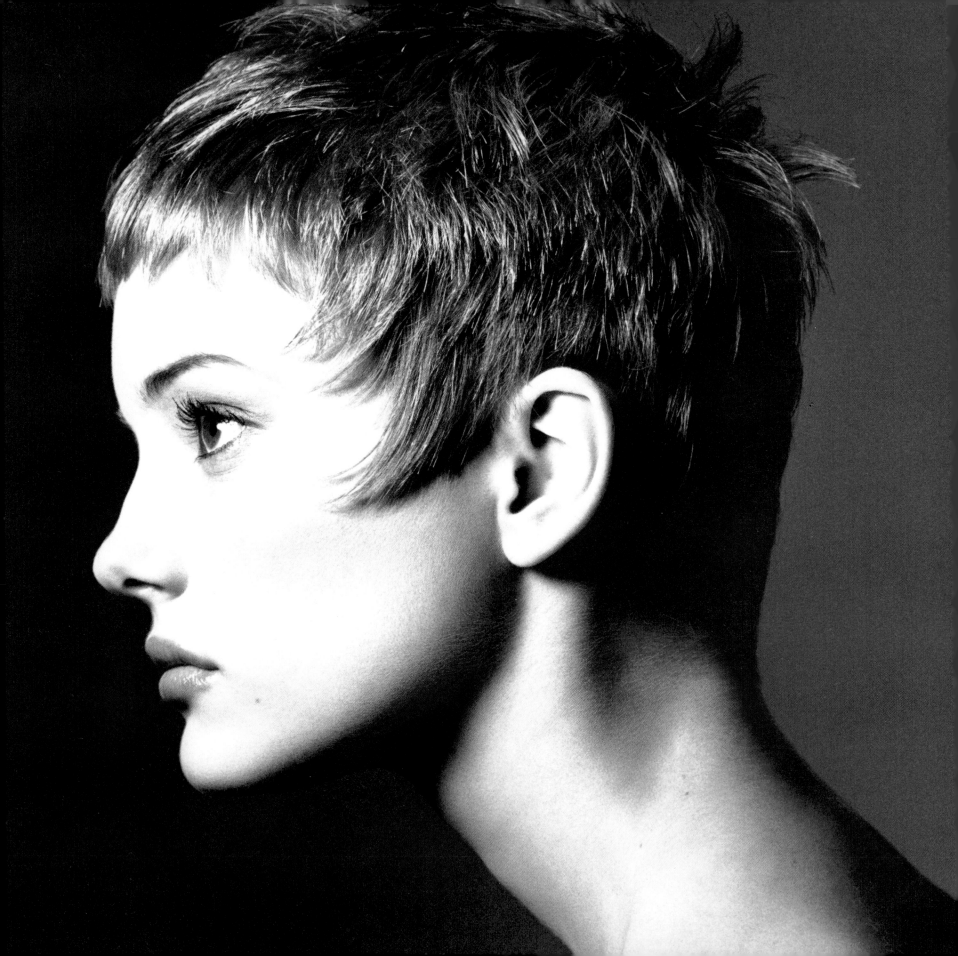

ease; if it's a coworker or friend, note if she has to make an extra effort to keep up the style (try to do this without looking like a stalker!). You should also see if you both share the same hair type, or ask if the stylist is successful with all kinds of hair.

If you don't get a good referral, which is the case a lot of the time, you'll be left to fend for yourself. But don't be afraid. There are plenty of ways to find a great stylist all by yourself. Regardless of where you live, you should have a good idea of where the best salons are in town. Make a list and call each one. The person you talk to will more than likely ask you generic questions about yourself, your hair, and what type of style/cut you're looking for. It's a good idea to give as much information as you can; it's all useful, and this will help the person determine which stylist is best suited to you. (This is also a good time to inquire about price.)

If the stylist is someone you've never met (and/or you know nothing about his or her work), you should consider setting up a consultation in advance of any actual appointment. It will give both of you the chance to see if you get along, not necessarily to see if you can be friends (although that's always a plus), but to see if you communicate well with each other and if you feel you can trust him or her with your hair. Before meeting, try to prepare answers to the following questions:

• What is your work life? Are you a homemaker, a professional, a student?
It's great to want to look good for yourself and others, either at home, at school, or at the office, but you really have to consider how full and busy your daily schedule is. Will you have the time (or the inclination) to work with a particular style, and is it going to be versatile enough to work in multiple situations and easy to style and care for on your own?

• What is your lifestyle? Are you active in sports? Do you like nightlife? Do you travel a lot?
If you're the type who's always on the go, then you may not have the time for an elaborate style. However, you may want to leave yourself some options for when you do slow down.

• Are you looking to be more sexy? Less sexy?
Of course, what *is* and what *isn't* is subjective, but a haircut can change the way people see you *and* the way you see yourself. So be prepared for a reaction if you go from long to short, straight to curly, or vice versa.

• Are you looking to make a drastic change? Small change? No change at all?
Be adventurous or not, but be willing to accept the results.

• How much time (and money) are you willing to put into the maintenance of a hairstyle?
Remember, in most cases, you do get what you pay for.

You might also refer to the style of a favorite celebrity or bring along pictures from magazines. Visuals are a great idea, but be prepared to hear that your choices might not be right for your hair type. (Also, as I've already said, a lot of things are created for pictures that are hard to duplicate in real life.)

Finally, try to arrive a bit early at the salon before your consultation to watch the stylist in action. You can see if the person is flamboyant and creative, or conservative and classic. Finally, if you are the least bit uneasy or uncomfortable with your meeting, remember that a consultation is not a commitment. You don't have to book an appointment afterward.

a cut above A combination of razors and notching and standard shears were used to create this simple but multidimensional short cut on Jaime Rishar, to the left. I think the style is feminine, edgy, *and* timeless. A favorite photo, courtesy of Troy Word.

the **shapes** of things to come

On these two pages, I put together five fundamental face shapes—oval, triangular, square, round, and long—plus information on head size (including neck and shoulders), with my recommendations on what to look for in an initial cut. I believe a good basic hairstyle will help you to not only look your best, but to change configurations with the same successful results. Also, a good cut can give you the "illusion" of movement or subtly change the shape of your face by layering the hair around the cheekbones, temples, eyes, and mouth. It's important to remember that I have also included some information on how coloring your hair through highlighting/lowlighting can further complement the look (and shape) of your face. Overall, you'll see that the basic premise behind what defines a good cut and good coloration is balancing your features. If a shape is top heavy, you counter it with something more on the bottom. If your face or your features (like the spacing of your eyes) is wide, you try to narrow the look with the way hair is placed and cut; if they are too narrow, you try to widen them, and so on.

Use the information as a starting place, but always keep in mind that if you are already comfortable and satisfied with the way you look, you shouldn't change things just because someone says so. However, you may end up liking something you hadn't considered by allowing yourself to be open to exploring new options. I also wish to make it perfectly clear that while the information is presented here in a somewhat lighthearted vein, I do not mean to imply that any particular face shape (or size) is more advantageous or attractive than another.

size

Your body type (both in weight and height) is the major factor in determining what size your face is. Interestingly, in beauty photographs, a model can have a small- or large-size head, but her face can appear ideally balanced because the body is often not visible for perspective and proportion. If you have what you consider a small head, something as simple as lift in front, along the top hairline, can give the face the illusion of more length. But don't overcompensate all over with enormous amounts of hair, as this will only make your head look as though it is in a bird's nest. On that same thought, avoid any hairstyle or cut that encroaches on the face, making it appear as though it is receding inward. For a large-size head, the reverse is typically true: Too much hair can make it appear even larger, and soft layering of hair around the face will help to make it look smaller. The shape of a haircut can also affect the look of your neck and shoulders: If you feel that your neck is unusually wide, a longer-length style to the shoulders, with layering, can make it seem narrower (be aware that very short cuts can make a thin neck look even skinnier). Hairstyles that are too wide across the shoulders will make them look small, and a cut that falls within them will make the shoulders appear wider.

oval

Typically, an oval is what one would consider the ideal facial shape. However, depending on the strength of your facial features, from cheekbones to the height of your forehead, etc., you may need to alter the shape of a cut (or style) by layering around the face to give it some more dimension and definition. Often bangs are a nice way to decrease the look of an overly oval shape, and since an oval can have a longish aspect, top-heavy styles tend not to be as successful because they can add too much elongation. **Color notes**: Darker coloring (lowlighting) all around the face will act as a soft frame to accentuate and define the oval shape.

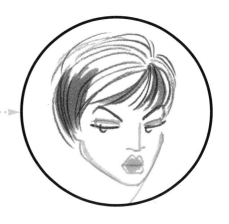

triangular

Also sometimes referred to as a "sweetheart" look because the face can resemble the shape of a heart. Distinguishing features: pointed chin and roundness above eye area. (A peak along the center hairline can accentuate the look.) The simplest cut to offset this shape is an inverted triangle, which will balance out the features. Avoid cuts that are top heavy, as this will only exaggerate the effect. Curly and wavy hairstyles will soften the often severe appearance of a triangular shape. **Color notes**: Highlight below the ears to widen the face, lowlight above the ears to narrow.

square

Squareness of the face, especially around the jawline, can give an individual the look of strength. However, it can be too stolid and hard-edged for some. Try layering around the face to soften your look. Additionally, curly and wavy styles are a great way to give the face some roundness. Normally, the length of a cut should extend below the jawline, or else the squareness of the face shape can become exaggerated. Furthermore, pulled-back or flattened hairstyles tend to shift the focus back to the jawline. **Color notes**: Soften the entire face by lightening the hair all around.

round

A round shape is usually equated with weight and/or added fleshiness of the face, often leaving it with softer or less-defined features. Soft layering of hair around the face will give it definition, but anything too geometric can make the shape look at odds with itself (e.g., circle in a square). Any cut, including curly or wavy styles, with width at the sides will likely make your face appear to be rounder. For this reason, one-length cuts to the shoulder are typically better than bobs. Also, try keeping curls back from the face, allowing loose, tousled pieces to frame and shape. Any extra fullness of a style on top of your head can make it appear more oval. **Color notes**: Try placing darker lowlights along the sides of the face to give it definition and lighter highlights at the top of the head to create length.

long

Long shapes tend to be easily exaggerated, however, the overall effect can be most striking if the style/cut is subtly defined by accentuating and layering of the hair around the face, especially at the cheekbone and eye areas. Wearing long, straight one-length hair will only further elongate your face, especially if the hair is darkly colored. Bangs are another good way to shorten the face, however, top-heavy hairstyles will, again, only add the look of more length. Cuts with more volume at the sides tend to widen the face and bring attention, in particular, to the eyes, and parting your hair to one side will create the look of more roundness, more than splitting it straight down the center. **Color notes**: Lighten up the sides of the face to create the illusion of more width and keep the forehead area darker.

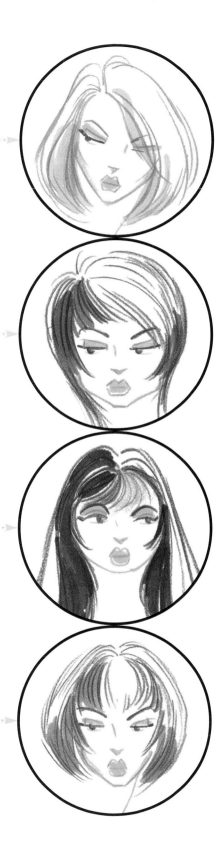

By this point, you should have a great haircut in a shade you adore, understand what can and *cannot* be done with your particular texture of hair, and know a little something about who you are and what to expect from your hair (and your stylist).

The following pages take you through the basic processes of cleansing, conditioning, texturizing and building, drying, styling, and finishing—a total of six different steps to a successful hairstyle. However, not everyone will have to undertake each process. You may be able to skip one or two, taking into account your own needs. And keep in mind that these steps work in tandem with each other, and one step does not necessarily stop completely before you begin the next; there is a great

prepare the hair

deal of overlap. Sometimes between texturizing and finishing, building and styling, it's hard to see where one process leaves off and another begins!

The information here should give you an idea of what to expect if you decide to change your current style or texture or if you just want to maintain your hair at its best the way it is.

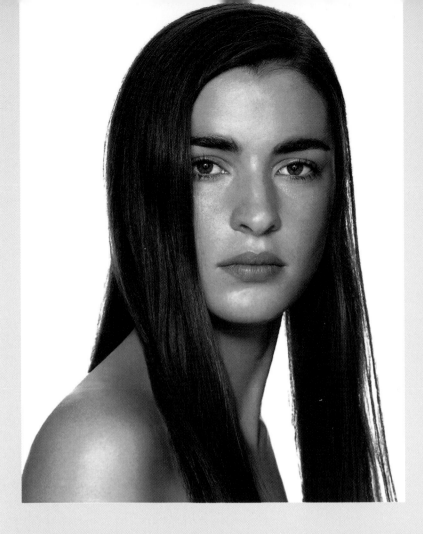

~ I was so happy we were able to get model Amanda Moore for the pictures on the next twelve pages. At the time she was shuttling back and forth between bookings in upstate New York and Malaysia. Luckily, we were able to squeeze her in between flights. She was a real trooper to go through the paces of posing for over a dozen pictures in only a few hours. Fortunately, we had the great photographer Troy Word at the helm to make sure every fleeting moment was captured on film.

I specifically wanted Amanda for these pictures because I think she looks extremely beautiful and accessible at the same time, which is actually a very rare quality in a model. Often they show up on the set looking less than ordinary, only to be transformed into a creature a bit too "out-of-this-world"–looking once all the primping and fussing is done.

To maintain healthy hair, you have to wash it regularly. However, that doesn't necessarily mean every day; you don't want to dry out your hair or your scalp. But it is important to "open up" the cuticle layer of each hair (which is what cleansing does) so that it can properly absorb conditioning and styling products. And a really good shampoo will get all the way down to the hair's roots and remove the oils, dirt, and buildup from other products without stripping or damaging the hair itself.

Shampoos typically come in four categories—dry, normal, oily, and chemically treated. You can also buy shampoos ranging from baby-fine to thick-hair formulas, with the former containing the least amount of emollients and the most detergents, and the latter containing just the

cleansing

opposite. (Emollients tend to weigh the hair down; avoid excessive amounts if you have limp hair.) Often you'll find that your hair is a combination of qualities, such as baby fine and color processed. In this case, I suggest that you use common sense in determining what formula your hair will most benefit from. (Remember, there is no law against using more than one shampoo at a time, in specific places, or using different ones on alternate days.)

soap story Lather does not clean your hair; it is mainly for show. In fact, I use a lot of European shampoos that hardly lather at all but do a great job of cleaning hair. However, keep in mind that the dirtier your hair is, the less it lathers, and the cleaner it is, the more suds you'll see.

73

You may have a combination of needs, like chemically processed hair that goes limp at the roots. You need to clean your scalp (and give it some lift), but you want to avoid stripping moisture from the rest of your hair. Before shampooing, apply a conditioner along the length of your wet hair to the ends (to act as a buffer). Then, when you're ready, concentrate the shampoo just at the root area, allowing only the runoff during the rinse to wash over the rest of your hair.

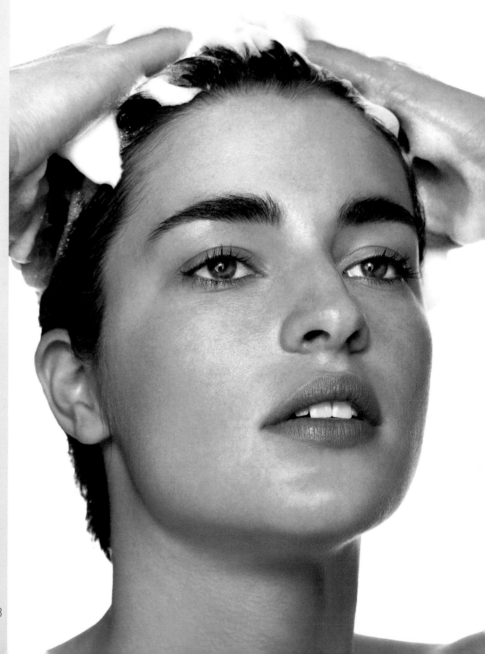

waterworld Cleansing and conditioning are wet processes, involving water from your shower, bath, or sink. Before you move on, you'll want to dry off a bit. Blot the hair gently with a towel, soaking up the extra moisture. Try not to *rub* the water out of your hair, as this will cause tangles. Leave some of the moisture in for texturizing, building, styling, and drying—which are all done in tandem. (If you have unusually thick hair, you can take a dryer and rid yourself of some of that extra wetness, but avoid blowing your hair around in all directions—what you'll end up with is a mess that will be impossible to get a brush or comb through and will cause unneccessary *stress* to your hair.)

grooms Grooms, including silicones, can be applied to damp or dry hair. Great for smoothing, taking the volume out, and adding definition to the hair texture (such as defining individual curls or chunks of hair).

Texturizing (and building) your hair may be a new concept for some, but it is simply knowing the natural quality of your hair—rough, silky, smooth—and reconfiguring it (if necessary) to suit your styling needs. To put it another way, working with hair today is not about re-creating an exact style, but about giving your hair a certain look. And

texturizing and building

whether that is tousled, slick, sexy, or innocent, it can be accomplished with the right texture.

Your hair's texture plays the leading part in successful styling. I like to think of texturizing and building as product layering, placing one on top of the other to build the ultimate individual texture. The keys to this process are knowing what styling result you want from your hair and utilizing the right products to achieve that. It might be helpful to think of it like applying foundation makeup: creating the best canvas to work upon. However, selecting texturizing and building products can be daunting with so many choices available. Even though hair care products are categorized by hair type and chemical processes to make choosing easier, finding the right ones will take a little trial and error. Stick with it until you do.

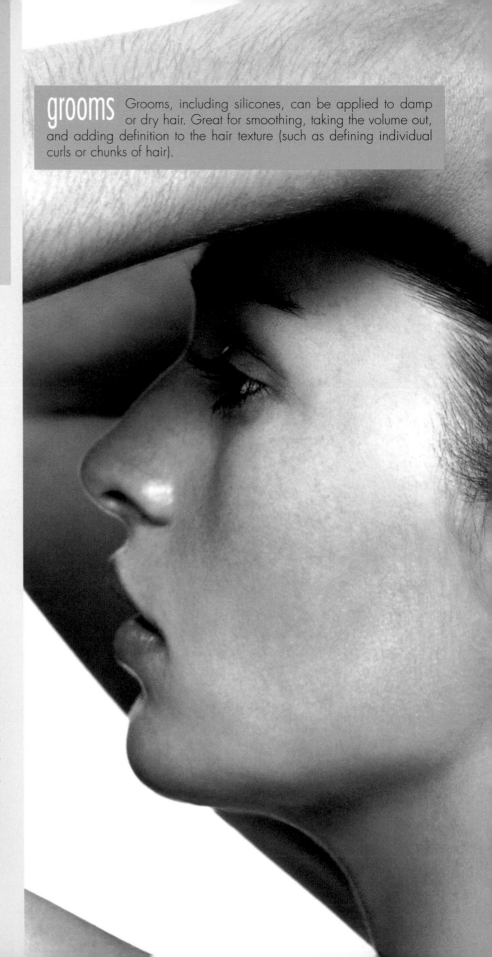

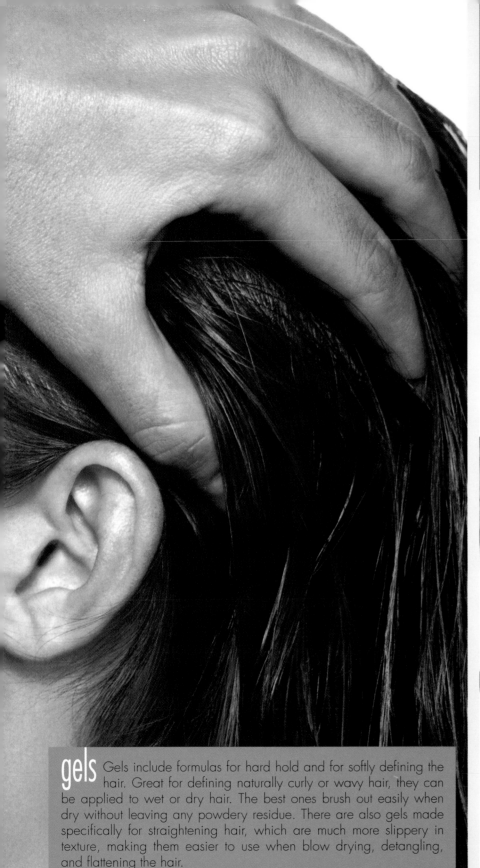

sprays

These include volumizing and styling (not holding or finishing) sprays and mousses. They are building products—designed to work on damp hair while it is being styled with a dryer and brush. Sprays can add body, provide rigid lift at the roots, and help configure (or reconfigure) hair into wavy and curly styles.

When applying spray (or for that matter any product used throughout this book) to hair, consider what your final styling goal is and target it accordingly. Do you need extra lift and support at the roots? Will you be curling or shaping the entire length of the hair? Is there a flip just at the ends?

1 Just at the roots
2 From the roots to midway, or midway to the ends
3 Just at the ends, or from roots to ends

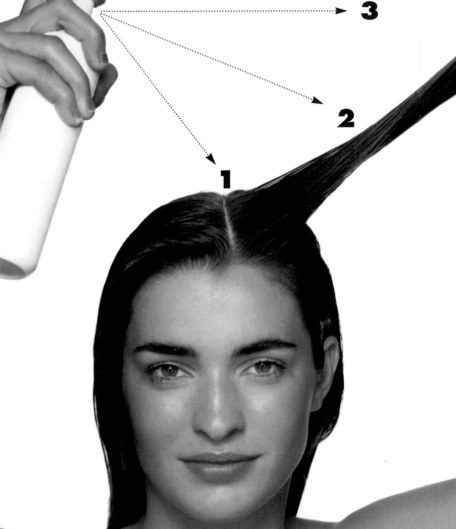

gels

Gels include formulas for hard hold and for softly defining the hair. Great for defining naturally curly or wavy hair, they can be applied to wet or dry hair. The best ones brush out easily when dry without leaving any powdery residue. There are also gels made specifically for straightening hair, which are much more slippery in texture, making them easier to use when blow drying, detangling, and flattening the hair.

clays

Clay grooms are not as common as other texturing and styling products, but I predict that will change, because they work extraordinarily well. Most are meant to be applied to hair that is already dry (as seen below). They work by holding hair together without the stickiness of other products, and they leave the hair with much more flexibility. They're also great for adding volume to fine, limp hair.

less is more

You don't need to use a lot of product in order it to be effective, even if you have enormous amounts of hair. Use it sparingly at first to see how much is really necessary.

This is a very simple and effective way to distribute product evenly.

the palm method

Place about a dime's worth of product in the palm of one hand. Gently put both hands together and rub in a circular manner, creating a thin film. (Be sure to confine the product to the inside of the palms and fingertips.)

Then you can either clasp sections of hair (as seen to the left), which keeps product evenly on both sides of the hair and away from the roots (this is a precise application, allowing more control over the placement of product, creating different levels of texture, volume, and direction of style), or you can run the fingers through the hair and onto the roots (see pages 76 to 77), for a more random, all-over application.

Whether you use a clay or creme groom, gel, or silicone, you can still apply product in the same three-step method described earlier, keeping in mind whether you need more or less support at the roots, the middle, and the ends. Also remember which products cut the volume of hair (silicones, creme grooms, gels) and which expand it (volumizing sprays, clay grooms).

styling · drying

Drying your hair entails much more than just getting rid of moisture; it's knowing when you are overdrying and how to properly use blow drying as a styling function itself. Remember, you can add to or reduce volume in your hair with a dryer; you can also straighten curly hair or give shape to straight hair, all depending on which tool you use with the dryer (from a simple comb through a myriad of different brushes).

A couple of other points: Typically, when drying and styling your hair from underneath, you are adding volume, shape, and/or lift (and using a brush). When skimming across the surface, you are generally smoothing and straightening (and often using a comb). However, the best way to straighten the hair is with a brush from underneath; gently pull the hair down in the direction it grows and apply intervals of hot and cool air with your dryer. Also, moving through the hair quickly with your dryer and brush (or comb) prevents overdrying or singeing the hair and creating unnecessary bumps or ridges.

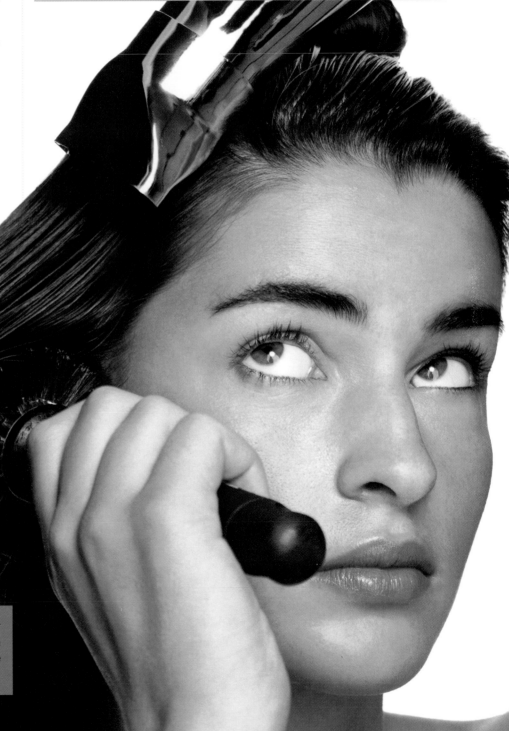

compression impression
The air compressor (nozzle) on your blow dryer works by concentrating the stream of air directly on the area where you are working. This prevents the air from blowing the hair around, creating flyaways, tangles, and over-blown hair. Always try to use yours.

round 'n' round
As you apply hot (and cool) air from your dryer, constantly twirling a round brush while moving it down the hair will not only keep the hair in place and on the brush, but accelerate the "polishing" action.

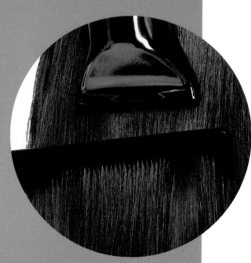

using a blow-drying brush

Using a blow-drying brush with your dryer is great for doing mainly these four things:

- Keeping the hair in control for overall drying
- Creating lift and support at the roots (as seen below)
- Redirecting the hair away from normal growth patterns
- General straightening

This is also a good brush to use (with your dryer) for simple one-step styling of straight to wavy hair into an easy shape like a bob.

using a comb

You can blow dry and style your hair using a comb. However, this is mainly a method used to straighten and smooth the hair. The subtle action of a comb running over and down the *outer* surface of the hair helps keep it under control. Follow the comb closely behind with a stream of hot air (be sure the comb is heat resistant). Then comb again, followed by a stream of cool air, to seal the cuticle layer. This will work even better if the hair has been treated with a silicone or straightening gel.

Note: Be aware that using a comb and a dryer will normally decrease the volume of your hair.

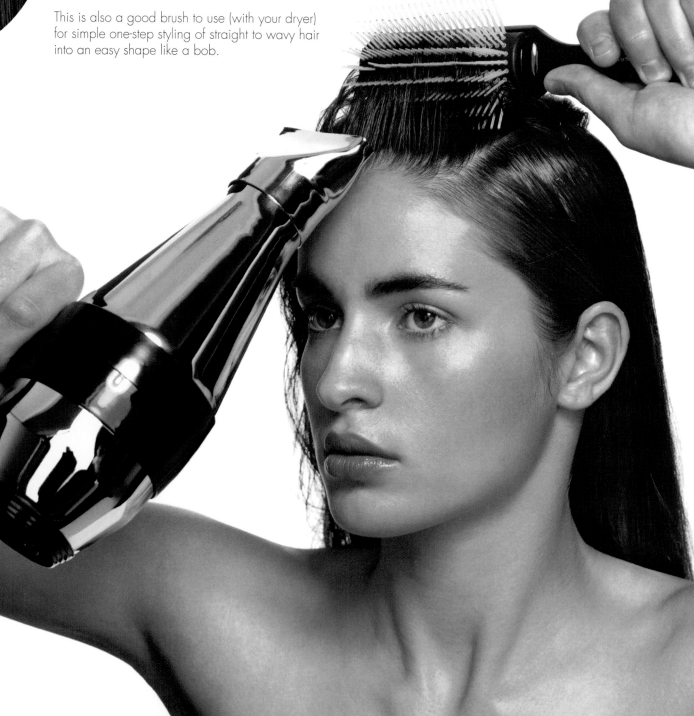

Obviously, curling your hair is not necessary for all hairstyles, but in this instance on Amanda, because her hair is very straight and very long, a little bit of curl was necessary to give it just the right amount of added waviness, volume, and movement.

My basic technique for curling hair with an iron is the same, regardless of the size of the curl desired. Your particular quality of hair will help determine whether or not you need to alter the level of application or use any particular styling product. **Note: Any time you use a hot appliance on your hair it's a good idea to protect it first. Try using a thermal styling spray or silicone; both create a slippery surface texture that also allows for faster and easier styling and, most important, prevents the iron from getting stuck in your hair.**

1 Decide the size of the curl and the direction it should go.

2 Turn on your iron and make sure it is placed in a safe spot (one where it is unlikely to be disturbed until you use it).

3 Section the hair into manageable pieces. Each piece should be brushed together and into a peak, then lightly spritzed with thermal styling spray.

4 Position the iron near the roots, open the clamp, and wind the hair around the barrel (making sure you are going in the right direction), leaving a bit of the ends sticking out. **Note: Sometimes the iron is too hot and can easily scorch the hair. I keep a spray bottle filled with water nearby that I lightly spritz on the barrel right before I use it to cool it down to a manageable temperature.**

5 With quick flexing movements, "pump" the clamp lightly, allowing the hair to move around the barrel as you wind in the excess hair and the ends. Move quickly, or else you may leave visible marks on the hair.

6 Allow the iron to set the hair for just a few moments, or only as long as is necessary for the desired curl. You don't want to singe the hair.

7 Gently open the clamp (just enough to release your hair, but not enough to unnecessarily expand the size of the curl) and pull the iron out sideways. Never pull down on the curling iron to get it out of your hair. It will likely get caught and pull out your curl.

8 Depending on the style, you can either release the curl and leave it hanging, gently tug on it (if you're going for a cascading effect), add a bit of silicone or clay groom to define it, pin it in place for a stronger curl, or slip it into a roller for an even stronger roller set.

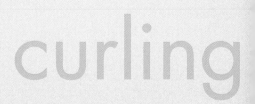

curling

no-fly zone

If you dry your hair against the direction it grows, you will increase the volume, but you can also increase the number of flyaways. (Try adding a touch of silicone or groom.) On that same note: Hot air creates more volume by opening the cuticle layer of your hair. Cool air closes it, making hair smoother.

style change

At the end of the day, your hair may have fallen in places. Instead of redoing the entire style, just take a blow-drying or round brush (and dryer) and try "spot lifting" at the roots. Again, on that same note: If you make a mistake with hair spray, don't fret. A light spritz of silicone to the area will dissolve the hair spray and allow you to rework it. You can also mist the hair with water and reactivate a product to freshen up a style, then blow dry.

keep it movin'

An unwanted "dent" or bend in the hair is usually created by allowing a brush to remain in one spot too long while the hair is cooling. Avoid this by keeping the brush moving down the length of the hair after the initial shaping is done.

a little extra

The added fullness and movement in Amanda's hair (to the right) was accomplished by combining the use of a large-barrel curling iron with a quick set on rollers. It's not always necessary to do it this way (especially if you have very voluminous hair already), but I find that the results are much more satisfying and longer lasting when the two are combined.

customize it

Sometimes products don't perform as well as manufacturers claim and will be successful only on specific hair types. But you have the ability to take these items and mix them together, creating custom blends that will function as well as you expect, or better. Combine volumizing spray with a bit of flexible spray to give you more flexible volume. Add a bit of silicone to your gel and make "gelicone." This makes the gel less sticky, so it goes on easier and gives you a softer hold. Try adding a bit of silicone to your creme groom, which can be heavy, and make "silicreme." You can also buy a fragrance-free shampoo and add a drop of your favorite essential oil (patchouli, jasmine, etc.), creating your very own scented hair cleanser.

weighing the options

A final note on products: Everything from grooms to gels is available in different weights and formulations. From spray silicones to creme grooms and pastes, it's hard to decide which one is right for your needs. There are a couple of rules of thumb: Normally, a spray formula tends to be the lightest-weight product and application, a paste is typically heavier (though that may just mean you need to use less of it). Cremes fall somewhere in the middle. Regardless of what you end up using, it's best to start out with a small amount and then add more product only if you're not getting the desired results.

In many cases, finishing is the simplest step and requires no more than brushing out the hair and topping it off with a light spritzing of holding or finishing hair spray. However, don't be fooled into thinking that that is the case in all instances. Sometimes you may want to control flyaways by adding a light layer of silicone or groom. If you have a curly or chunky style, this is the time to separate curls and pieces of hair, giving them definition. The point is to make the extra time (which might only be a moment or two) and effort to add your own personal "signature" to your hair the way the best hairstylists do. I'm sure you've noticed that they will snip and clip up to the last minute you're in the chair. It is not obsessive behavior. They're giving your hair the individual touch that gives it character.

finishing

~ When it comes to beauty pictures (or commercials, for that matter), wind is frequently used to create just the right touch of movement. That was the case with this final portrait of Amanda. But we're not talking gusts of wind, only a slight breeze from a small handheld fan. What it does, aside from the obvious, is to take the image out of the category of an ordinary beauty portrait. With the right lighting it also allows the hair to reflect highlights, giving it even more fullness.

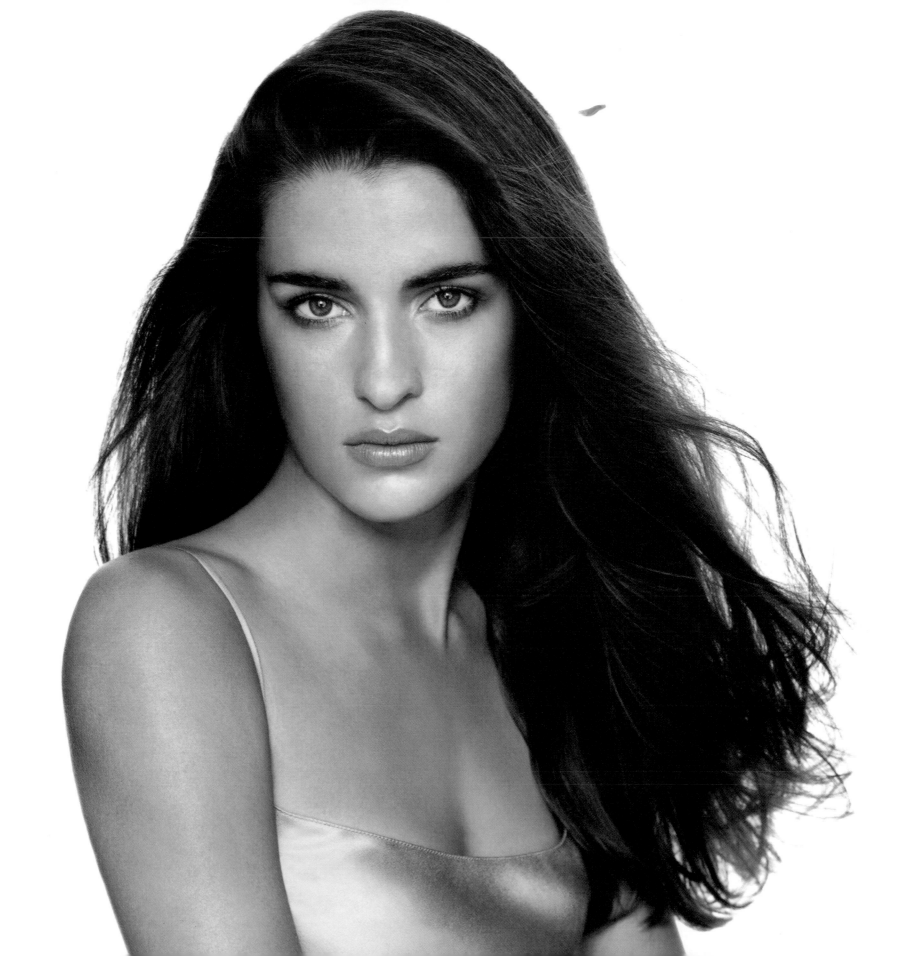

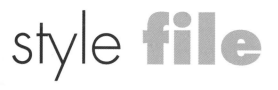

work with it Gorgeous Stephanie Seymour (right) is rarely seen with her hair styled in such a wild and sexy way as this, but I knew I wanted the look for at least one of her two pictures (the second is on page 101). What you might not be aware of is that her hair is very close to this normally. I don't mean unruly, but the texture, naturally, has a lot of movement, wave, and body. All I did was apply a bit of creme groom and separate, twist, and define random sections of hair. Then I applied hot air to her hair (turned upside down) with a diffuser for extra lift at the roots. Right side up, I defined a few more pieces (some had "broken" apart) and just had fun roughing it up. While it might be time-consuming to get just the right look and amount of implied movement, this style is not difficult to achieve. Just work with it.

style file

One of the misconceptions about hair care is that you cannot duplicate at home what is created in a salon. This is simply not true. Certainly some styles and techniques tend to be more difficult than others, but given enough instruction and patience, you can become a "master of your own mane." I find that more often than not, it really comes down to a question of time; you either have it, or you don't (so you won't bother). Given the overcrowded lives we all live, "wash-and-wear" styles have seemed the only way to go. But fear not, between advances in chemical formulas and processes, and the availability of information in books like this, it is easier than ever to achieve professional results on your own.

Many of the faces you'll see in this chapter will be familiar to you, and it is with great pleasure that I present them here (and throughout the book). I made a deliberate attempt to select images that would give you a variety of different styles and textures to look at, enjoy, and, if the mood hits you, try for yourself. I also made an effort to show looks on each person that were (slightly to wholly) different from how you would normally see him or her. You may not find an exact match (hair color, cut, or texture), but you should be able to find something that attracts you. When you do, take some time to assess your own tresses, and remember that a given hairstyle may need some alteration to be successful on you. That could entail something as simple as a bit more support (or conditioning) at the roots, or a bit more "polishing" (or volume) at the ends. Note: The step-by-step instructions that accompany each style were written as though they were being told to the subject of the picture. However, even if you are not a perfect length or texture match to the person in the photo, you should still be able to apply much of the information to the styling of your own hair.

Stephanie Seymour, photographed by Don Flood

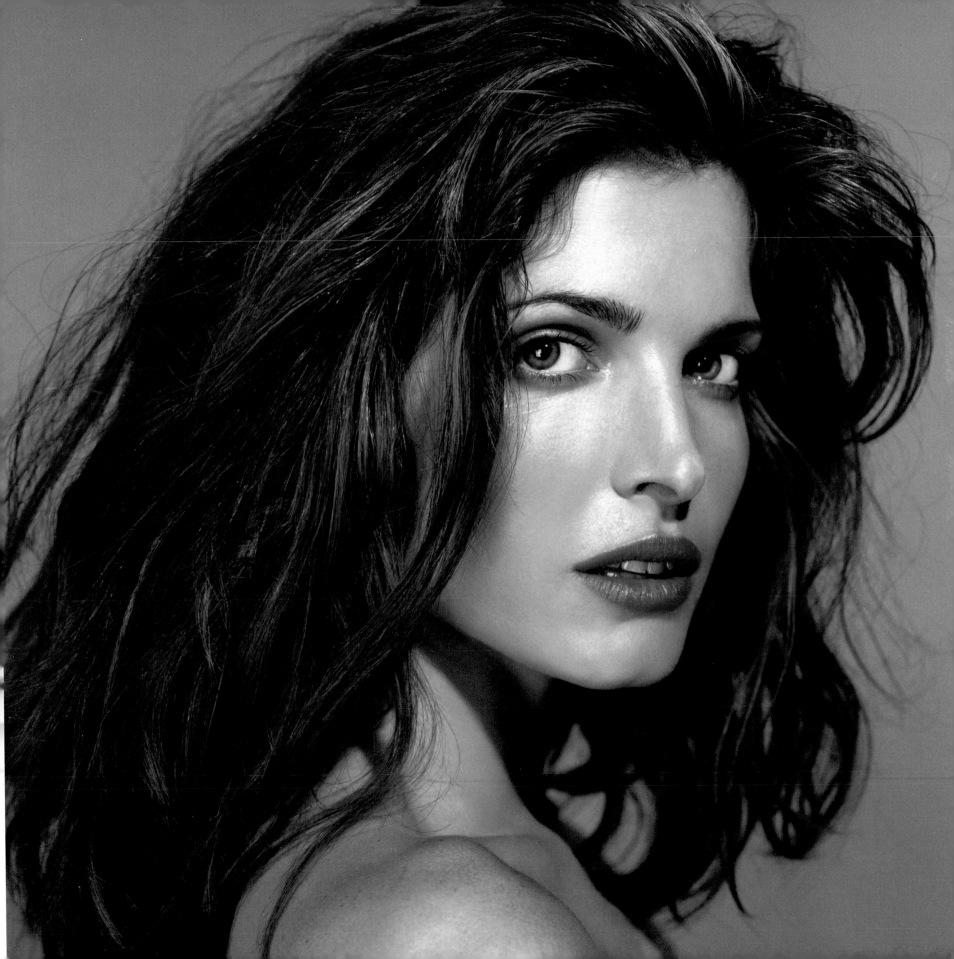

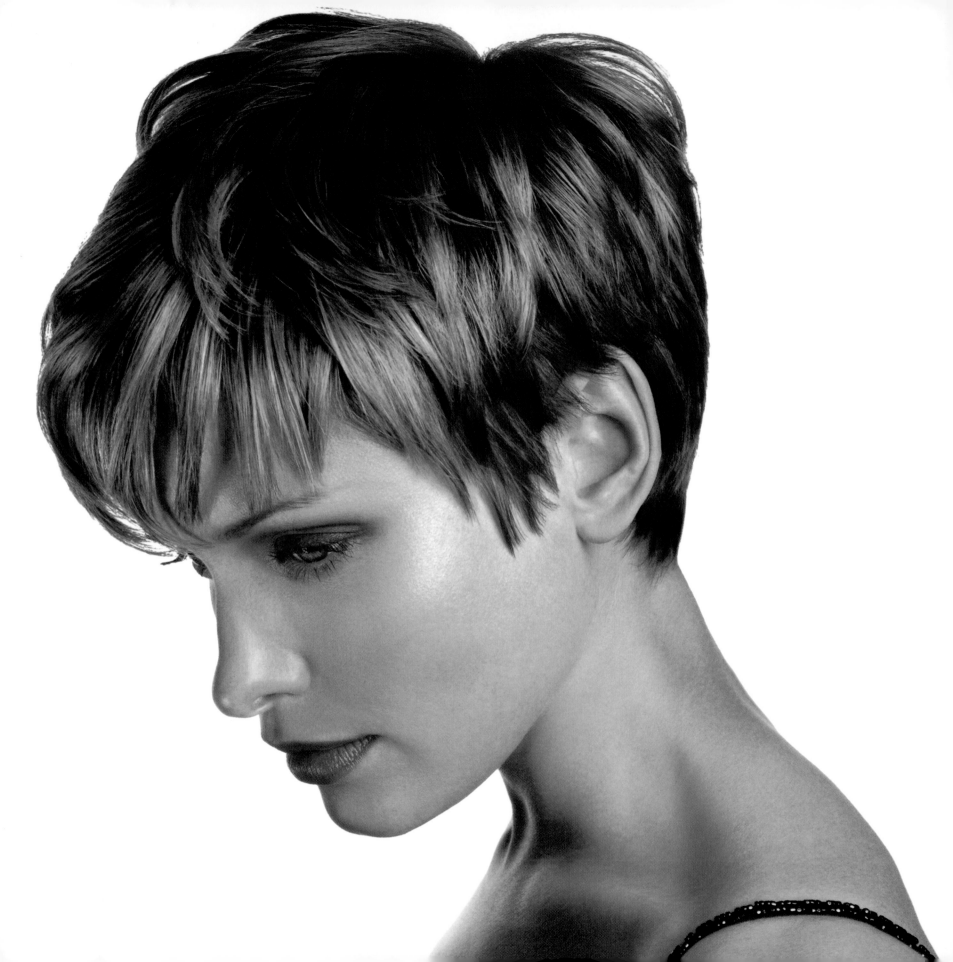

jenny

hair type: normal, medium thickness with a slight bend
special process: mix of pale and golden blond highlights
cut: short sides and back; longer layering on top

tools

blow dryer with compressor
blow-drying brush • small flat-plate ironing tongs (optional)

products

shampoo (for normal hair) • reconstructing conditioner
flexible styling spray (or soft-hold mousse) • clay groom

For this picture, Jenny's hair was highlighted to add more texture and brightness. Uneven "chunky" layers were made in the hair using standard shears, and the ends were thinned to create a head-hugging shape.

1 Shampoo, rinse, and towel blot.

2 Condition for about five minutes, rinse, and blot with towel.

3 Spray on styling spray or apply mousse at the roots, with a lighter application to the ends.

4 Begin drying your hair *without* a brush to see what happens. You might be surprised at the beautiful texture that occurs naturally. (If you have a great cut and the hair is responding well, and you want a "rougher" look, this can be a quick alternative styling method, allowing you to skip the brush and tong steps.) If not...

5 Using your blow-drying brush, blow and brush your bang area first, then work with the natural "bend" in the hair, give it a lift at the roots and blow out in multiple directions.

6 When hair is completely dry, rub clay groom into a film in the palms of your hands and apply it to hair while separating layers and pieces into exaggerated chunks.

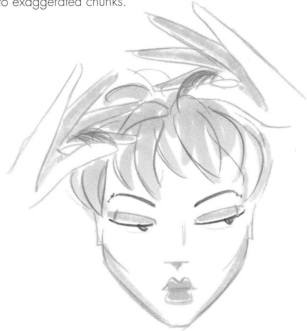

Optional: Iron the ends of each separated piece, concentrating mainly on the bang area, to give them more definition. (The iron should not be tightly clasped against hair, flattening it. Allow a little give to gently curve the hair to the ends.)

No hair spray should be necessary to finish this look, since the style will change and get better looking as the day and evening progress. Texturing your hair this way, first by highlighting, then using styling aids, can set up your hair for hours of accidentally beautiful changes. Just put your hands through it, move it around, and see for yourself. That's all I did!

cover girl Maybe you don't recognize her from this picture, but our lovely "Clipper" girl is also our beautiful cover model. For the cover look, which was done after this one, Jenny's hair was blown free of any curl, even the slightest bit of movement, and a generous amount of creme groom was added in. Then, with a fine-tooth comb and a blow dryer, her hair was flattened against the scalp even more. Finally, with the same comb (and my fingertips), I sectioned the hair into chunks along the front hairline, creating a sculpturally shaped bang. Because I used groom instead of gel, the hair is actually much softer to the touch than it appears. Incidentally, both shots, and the trio of images on page 55, were taken on the very same day.

arch 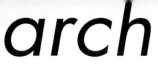 rigid roots to midshaft; soft, flexible ends

melissa

hair type: baby fine and straight (and a lot per square inch!)
special process: light blond foil highlights
cut: long layers with low-angled front

tools
wide-tooth comb • blow-drying brush
blow dryer with compressor and diffuser • (large) round brush
medium- and large-sized self-sticking rollers • styling clips
finishing brush • bobby pins (ridgeless)

products
shampoo (for baby-fine, highlighted hair)
reconstructing conditioner (for bleached hair)
volumizing spray • flexible styling spray
silicone • clay groom

Melissa's hair was highlighted with lighter tints of blond to give it the look of movement while adding pliability and volume for styling.

1 This first step is necessary for those with moderate to severely dehydrated or damaged hair. Apply reconstructing conditioner to dry hair (about four inches from roots to the ends) and leave on for a few minutes. Shampoo normally. Blot with a towel and reapply reconstructor to the same place and comb through. Leave for a few minutes, rinse, and blot with towel. (Be gentle. Do not rub the hair dry, as this will cause tangles.) Comb with wide-tooth comb.

2 On damp hair, concentrate volumizing spray on the roots, then lightly spray all over.

3 Spray hair lightly with flexible styling spray to help hold the bend.

4 Smooth a very small amount of silicone on hair from midshaft to ends. (For this texture hair, you need only a very light application of silicone to produce an easy brush-glide blow dry.)

5 Take a large section of hair in back, from ear to ear, and pin to the top of your head. Begin drying hair with blow-drying brush, gently pulling hair downward. When section is dry, switch to large, round brush and smooth ends. Repeat this section by section until you reach the top.

6 At the top, exaggerate the drying effects by pulling the hair forward and up, for lift. Again, switch to round brush and repeat until hair is smooth and shiny.

7 Take medium-sized rollers and set the hair on top in the same way that you dried it—directing them forward—adding a light spritz of styling spray to each roller (being careful not to actually wet them). Clip if necessary.

8 Set the back of the hair using approximately four large rollers, being careful to include the hair from the sides.

9 With the diffuser attachment in place, pass blow dryer over rollers for about five or six minutes, letting them cool while you do your makeup.

10 As each section is taken off rollers, smooth on a very light application of clay groom.

11 Brush hair with a finishing brush.

12 Pull sides back and fasten with bobby pins (you can use a bit more clay groom on the sides to help with pliability). Let hair from above fall over top of pinned hair.

13 Take a section of the hair on top, from the forehead back (being careful not to disturb the sides), and brush forward. Split this section in two horizontally. Brush the newly created back section straight up, and back comb lightly at the root. Brush out the front of this section of any back-combed hairs. Let go and brush back. Repeat this process with front section, and spritz with light holding spray.

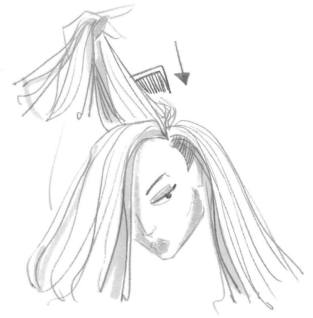

Melissa Brown, photographed by Don Flood

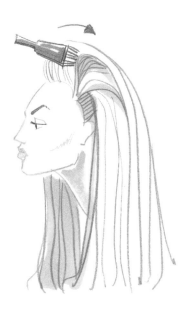

Is this you? Do you hate your fine, flat tresses so much that you think it's okay to use a bar of soap on your delicate hair just because it turns out so full? Don't do it. For the most part, bar soap is very drying and will only hurt your hair. Just shampoo normally and use a conditioner afterward. You'll be surprised at how responsive your hair will be. Remember that moisture (from a compatible conditioner) will give your hair softness *and* flexibility —two things that help hair to curl and move.

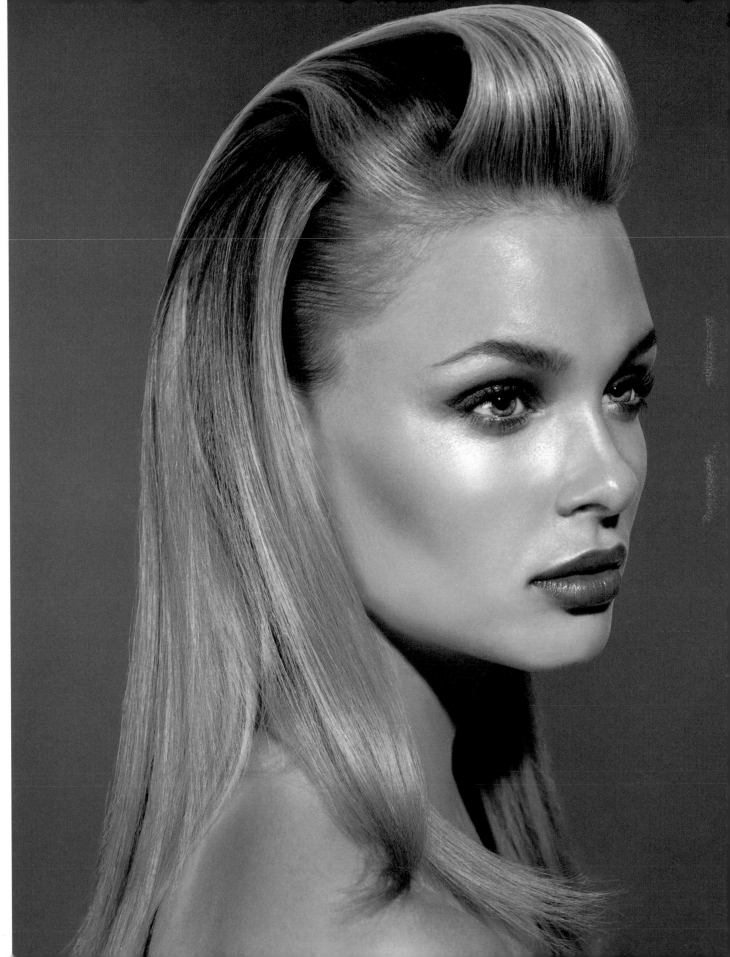

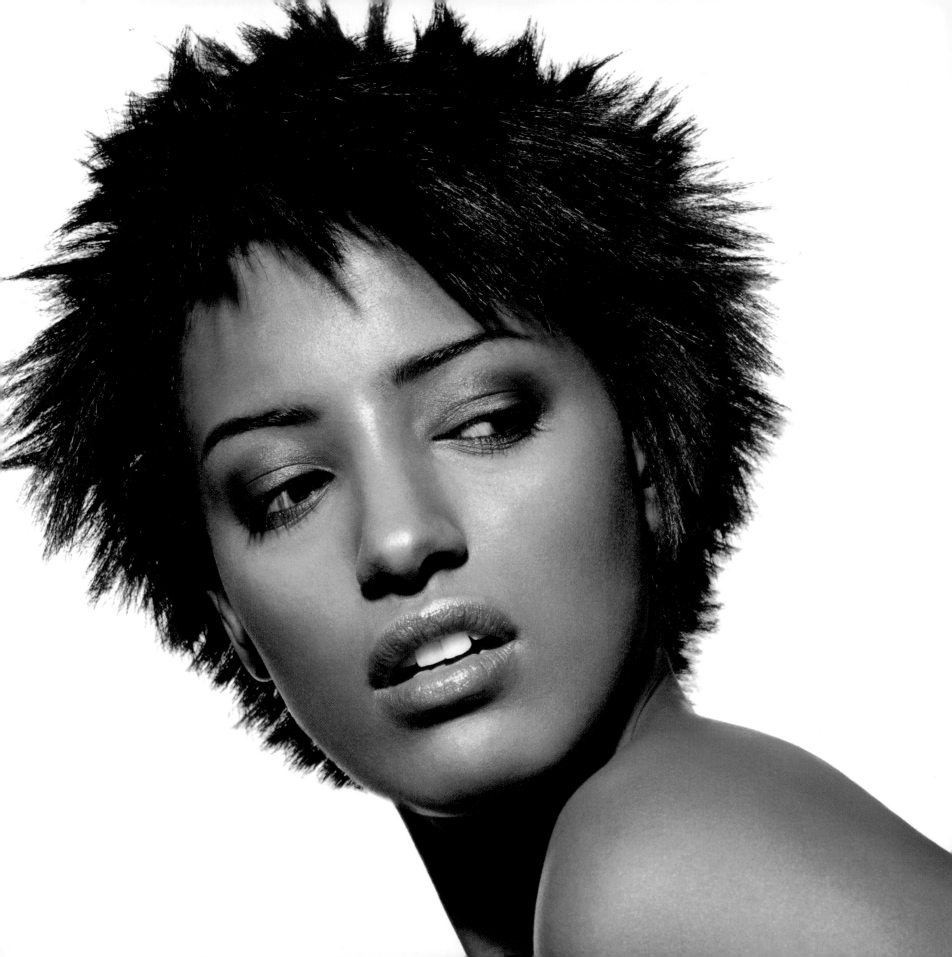

ella

hair type: thick, coarse, and curly
special process: relaxed
cut: short, layered diamond shape

tools

hard rubber comb • blow-drying brush
blow dryer with compressor • straightening tongs
fork comb

products

shampoo and conditioner (for chemically treated or dry, damaged hair)
conditioner (for softening) • straightening gel
creme groom • light holding spray

Because of the short length of Ella's hair, it was relaxed to open it up, not necessarily to straighten it, which could leave it looking too flat. Incidentally, if Ella's hair were dried naturally, it would look like a shorter version of Halle Berry's (on page 110), but with a looser curl.

1 Shampoo.

2 Comb first conditioner through hair and leave on for at least five minutes (or as long as the manufacturer suggests), rinse, and blot with towel. Apply second conditioner in same manner, rinse, and towel dry well. (These steps are good for anyone with chemically processed hair.)

3 Rub straightening gel into palms and apply to hair.

4 With dryer set at a high heat–high volume airstream, begin blow drying the hair (with compressor in place), using the hard rubber comb to move the hair forward first, then in every direction. (Make sure to follow every stroke immediately with the dryer.) Combing can be a bit rough at times, but the tension it creates is good for straightening. (A tip: Push the comb along with the dryer, moving fast so as not to burn the hair.)

Note: When hair is dry, it should look like an unfinished version of the photograph to the left.

5 Place a dime-sized amount of creme groom in the palm of your hand and rub palms together to create a film. Then, as though you are passing your palms across the edge of a paintbrush's bristles, lightly apply to hair. With remaining product, "comb" through hair with your fingers, pressing creme into the hair as you go along.

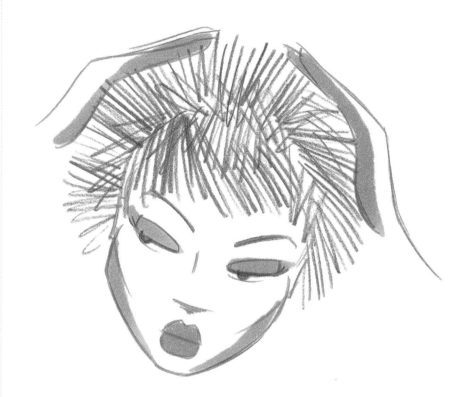

6 Using your comb, take small sections of hair at a time and press hot straightening tongs from about halfway up the hair shaft to the ends, leaving the other half unpressed. (The unpressed roots will support your style. If you flatten this area too, you may end up with a "flat" hairstyle, and you will need to use a lot of spray to get the hair to stand up.)

7 Loosely style with fork comb.

8 Finish with a light overall spritz of holding spray.

Ella Thomas, photographed by Nicolai Grosell

zigzag rigid roots; flexible from midshaft to ends

This is the kind of style where the more hair you have the longer it will take, but the more fantastic the results will be, as you can see on beautiful model Angie Hsu.

1 Shampoo, rinse, and towel dry.

2 Comb conditioner through hair with a large-tooth comb (to detangle). Rinse and towel dry.

3 Apply styling spray all over hair from roots to ends, adding a bit of silicone just at the ends, up to about three inches.

4 Assuming that your hair was already stick straight when you began, gently dry it with a blow-drying brush, following each stroke with the dryer.

5 When the hair is completely dry, check to see if the ends are thick and bristly. If they are, "polish" them smooth with a large round brush.

6 Beginning in the back, take large sections of hair and pin up on top of your head. Using your fingers, remove smaller sections of hair (a bit smaller than crimping plate) from the pins and hold them straight with light tension. Take the iron, lined up horizontally to the roots, and press firmly. Hold for a few seconds and move down the length of the hair, being careful not to disturb already-crimped hair. Continue until entire head is done, leaving a few straight, uncrimped pieces in the front. *See illustration opposite.*

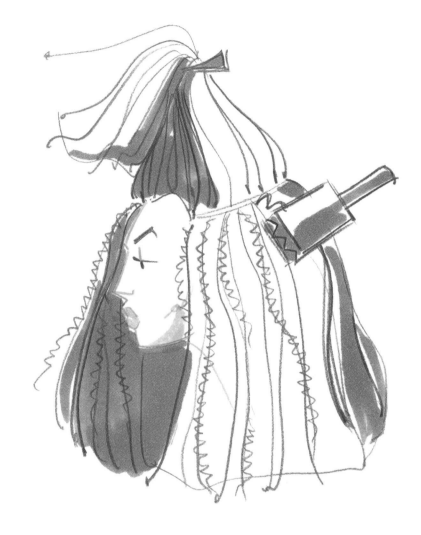

7 When crimping is complete, finger comb thickening groom through the hair. This will open up the hair and give it more volume. The more you work it, the more voluminous it will become.

Note: This style can be brushed, but I suggest doing so from underneath the hair to preserve the definition of the outer layer.

Angie Hsu, photographed by Don Flood

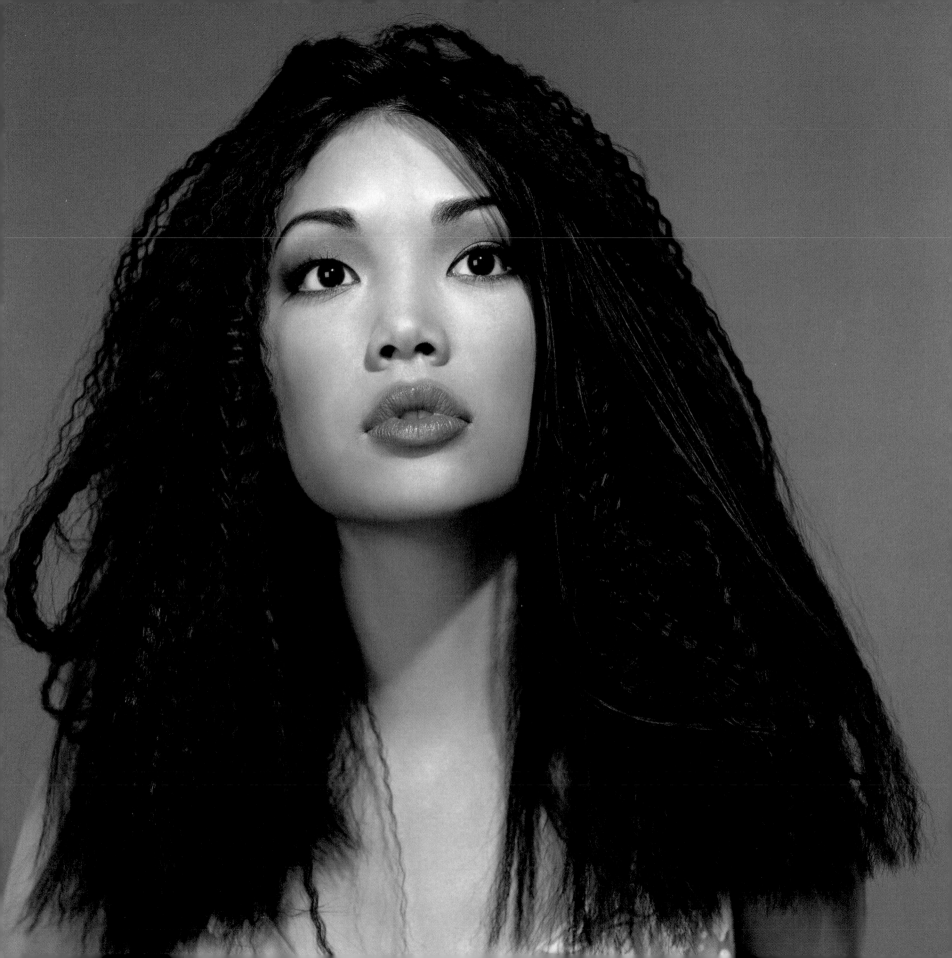

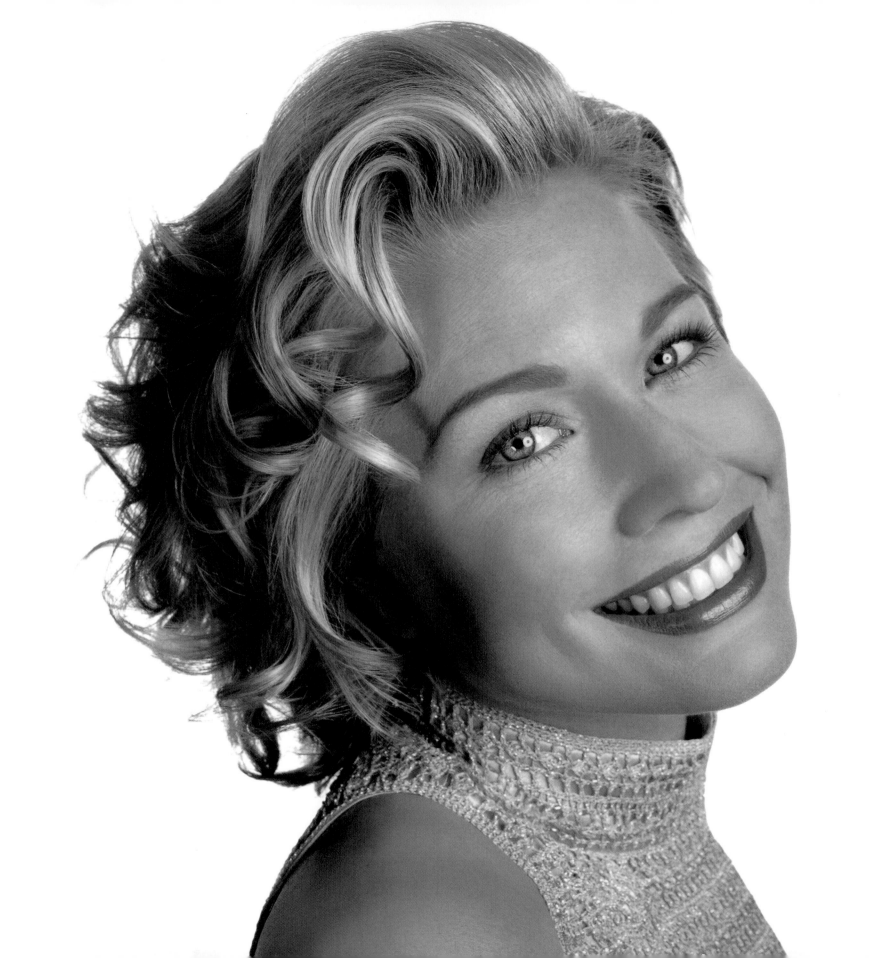

emme

hair type: straight and fine
special process: ash blond highlights
cut: midlength layers with long bangs

tools
large-tooth comb • blow dryer with compressor
blow-drying brush • (medium) round brush
medium-barrel curling iron • pin clips • finishing brush
fork comb

products
shampoo (for gentle, deep cleansing or chemically treated, fine hair)
reconstructing conditioner
lightweight softening formula conditioner (for the ends)
volumizing spray or extra-volume mousse • medium-hold styling spray
creme thickening groom • clay groom (optional)

Remember what I said earlier about how a hairstyle should frame the face? A perfect example of that sentiment is this portrait of lovely Emme Aronson. With such a gorgeous smile and twinkling eyes, I deliberately kept the curls back and away from her winning features. Incidentally, for the picture, Emme's hair was given a foil highlighting to texturize the hair, making it more pliable and easier to style.

1 Shampoo.

2 Comb reconstructing conditioner through hair and leave on for at least five minutes (or as long as the manufacturer suggests). Rinse, then squeeze out excess water. Apply softening conditioner to the ends, leaving on for about one minute. Rinse and blot with towel.

3 Use blow dryer to remove excess moisture, but do not dry hair.

4 Apply volumizing spray (or mousse) starting at the roots up to about one-half the length of the hair. Then spray entire head with styling spray. On the ends, apply a small amount of thickening groom.

5 Across the back of the head (from ear to ear), pin up the top half of your hair. Dry and smooth the bottom half.

6 Release the top section and continue drying, lifting for more volume at the roots. Blow, dry, and "lift" in all directions, up and back, working your way toward your forehead.

7 Use the round brush to polish the ends and give them a strong *backward* direction. However, do not overdry.

8 Section hair (as in the drying step) and begin curling hair in back in small sections. The pattern you use is not important. Release the top half and continue working your way to the front. Here, you'll want to direct the curls in a pattern moving away from the part and down the sides. Pin clip each curl.

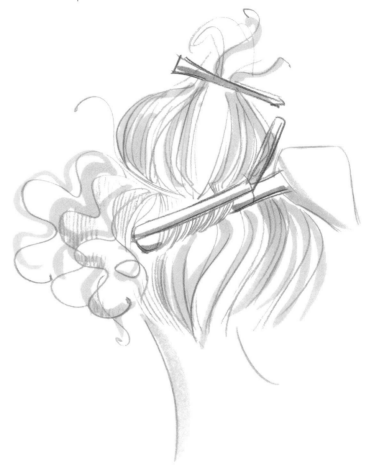

9 When finished, release all the curls and shake your head, combing through with your fingers. Use the finishing brush to smooth and direct hair in front. (You may want to use a little clay groom to contour rough spots into smooth waves. But use it sparingly, otherwise you'll weigh the hair down.)

10 Do a little back combing in front for extra lift and position hair with a fork comb. Smooth over with a finishing brush.

11 Finish off with a light once-over using the medium-hold spray.

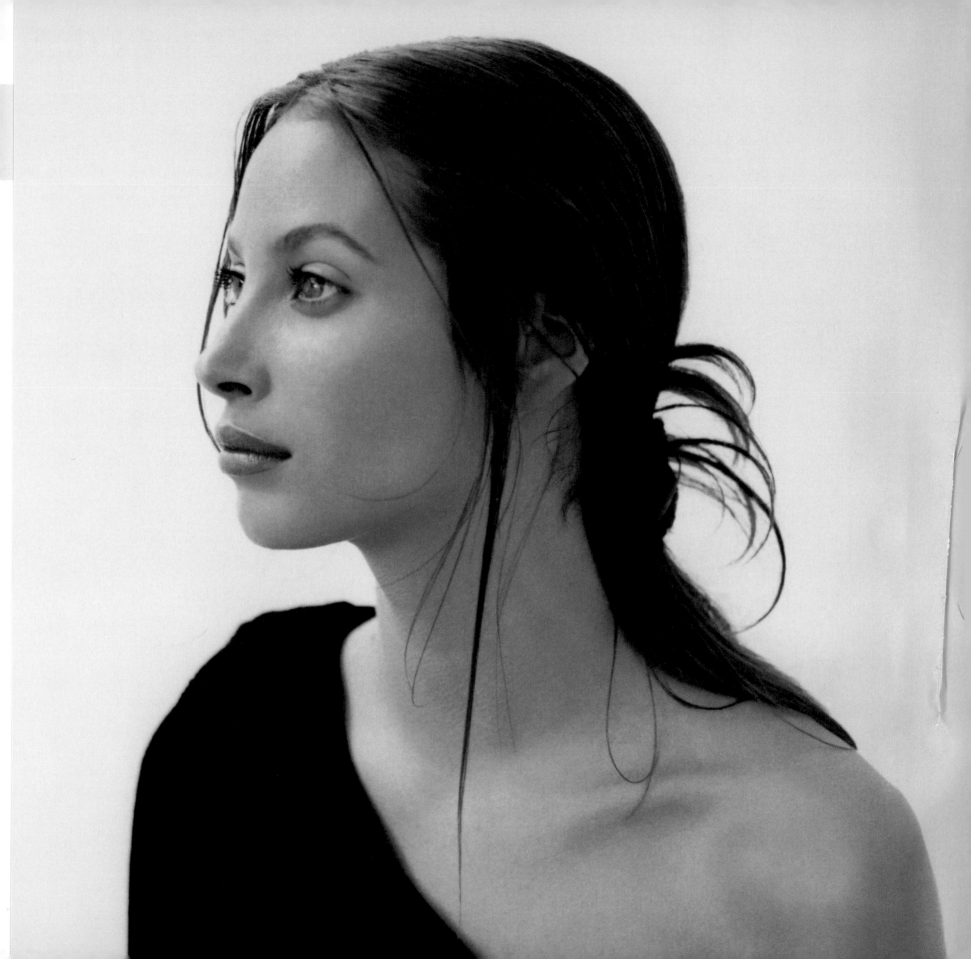

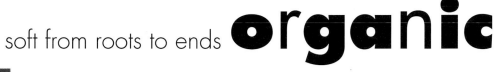

christy

hair type: curly, medium coarse
special process: none
cut: one-length back with low-angled layered front

tools
large-tooth comb • blow-drying brush
blow dryer with compressor • (large) round brush • paddle brush
large U-shaped pins

products
shampoo and softening conditioner (for dry hair)
straightening gel • silicone • clay groom • styling spray

Christy Turlington is a fashion muse who has inspired designers and photographers alike (not to mention a few hairstylists) to create extraordinarily beautiful things, like this sitting with master lensman Patrick Demarchelier for *Harper's Bazaar*. Another version became that issue's cover.

1 Shampoo, rinse, towel blot.

2 Apply conditioner and comb through, leave on for one to five minutes (depending on need), rinse, towel blot.

3 Apply straightening gel to entire length of hair. Comb through and add a touch of silicone to the ends.

4 Section hair across back of head and pin top section up.

5 Using the blow-drying brush, straighten hair with dryer on high heat. When hair is almost dry, switch to round brush to polish hair smooth. Do this, section by section, until hair is completely dry.

6 Add clay groom in sections (see the "palm method" described on page 78), and brush through.

7 With paddle brush, gather hair together in back to make a low ponytail, dropping out pieces on both sides to hang in front.

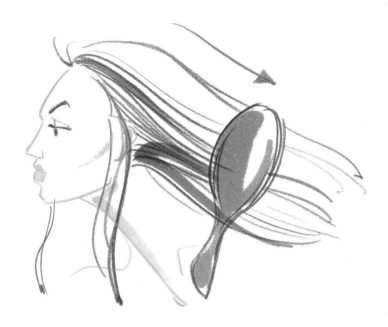

8 Take ponytail and twist against nape of neck, fastening low underneath with pins.

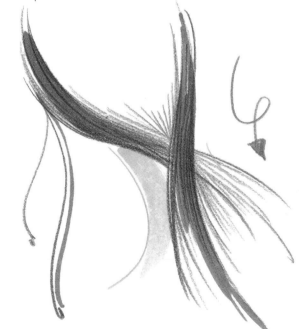

9 Pull out a few sprigs of hair and spray into place.

Christy Turlington, photographed by Patrick Demarchelier for Harper's Bazaar

slide soft and flexible from roots to ends

stephanie

hair type: wavy, medium coarse
special process: caramel brown highlights
cut: long layers; low-angled front

tools
wide-tooth comb • tail comb • blow-drying brush
blow dryer with compressor • (large) round brush • finishing brush
flat iron (optional)

products
shampoo (for dry hair) • reconstructing conditioner
straightening gel • clay groom • holding spray

This simple, straight style is a big transformation for Stephanie Seymor, who normally wears her hair with a smooth, wavy texture. It also subtly changes the way the shape of her face looks (check out page 85). Also notice that the long layering adds movement when the hair is worn natural (in the earlier picture), but disappears when the hair is straight, as it is shown here.

1 Shampoo with a dry-hair formula and lightly towel dry.

2 Condition, using a wide-tooth comb to detangle the hair. Rinse and blot.

3 Section and lift the hair using the tail end of a tail comb (or your fingers, if you like), to expose roots for application of straightening gel. (Use a light application at first, from roots to ends, then increase amount only if needed.)

4 With your head upside down, begin drying and brushing the hair in every direction (using a blow-drying brush quickly followed by the blow dryer set at high heat). With your head up, take sections of the hair (beginning at the back of the head), pulling down with the blow-drying brush and drying with airstream going in the direction of the hair growth. Once you've gone over the entire head, change to the round brush and go over the hair again, brushing and blowing until the hair is shiny and smooth.

5 Apply clay groom to "finish" the hair and use the finishing brush to keep the hairs together and control flyaways at the part.

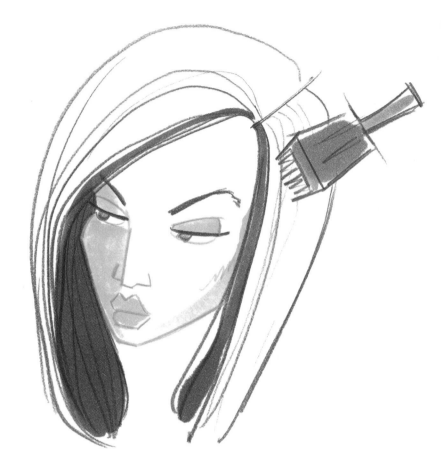

6 To hold, spray lightly with holding spray.

Optional: For further straightening, use a flat iron.

call of the curl
Since ancient Egyptian times, women (and to some degree men) have associated curly hair with supreme attractiveness. Because of this, many women throughout history went through the most extreme measures to get it, using things as dangerous as metal rods heated over an open fire and primitive pomades (made with animal fats and glues) to hold a curled set in place. As improbable as it sounds in this age of straightening and relaxing, the truth is it really wasn't until the latter part of the twentieth century that people began to covet straight hair.

Stephanie Seymour, photographed by Don Flood

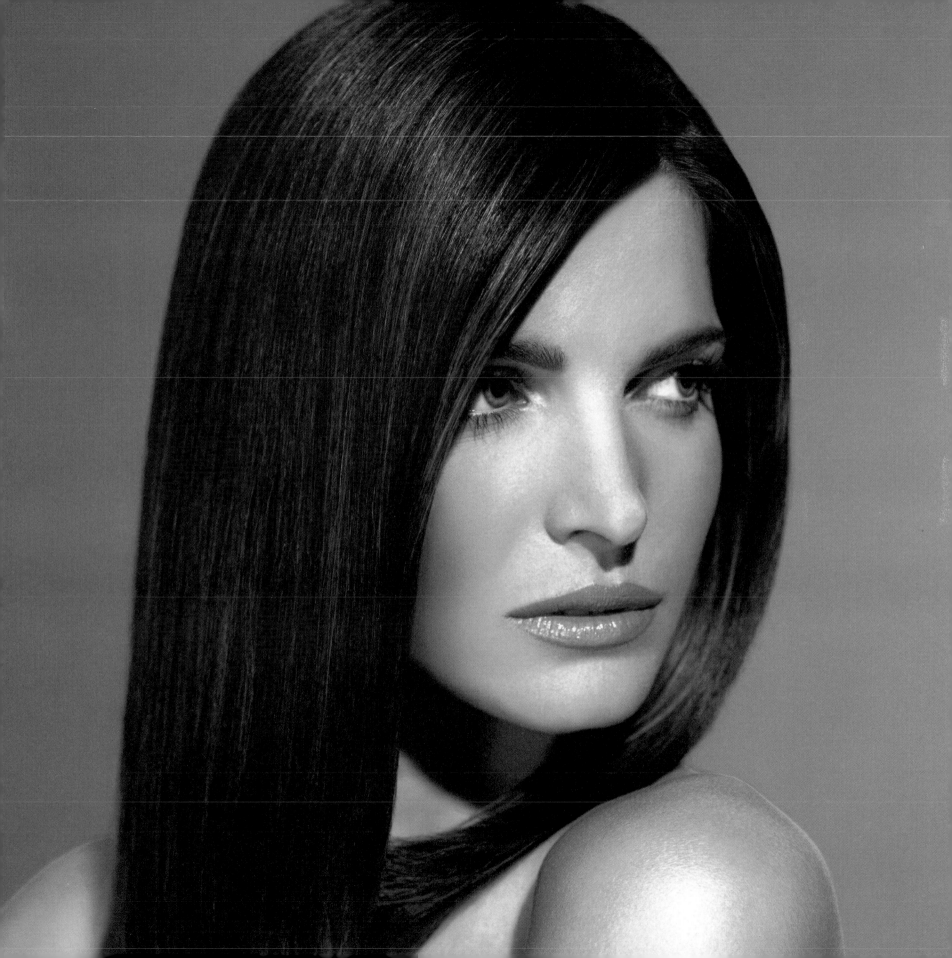

easy rigid roots and ends

a. j.

hair type: thick and wavy
special process: none
cut: short and uneven (to match contours of head and natural movement of hair)

tools
blow dryer with diffuser (optional)

products
shampoo and conditioner (for normal hair) • gel

Let's face it; guys want a no-nonsense haircut that needs little or no maintenance. They want to shower in the morning, wash their hair, condition it (once in a while), dry it, and go. And whereas women understand the concept of the use of multiple hair products, most men don't. To them it's just not necessary, and in most cases I'm inclined to agree. A. J.'s a perfect example of a great-looking guy who really only needs to attend to his hair with minimal effort to look fantastic. If you're one of the lucky ones, the following basic men's grooming steps should already be familiar.

1 Shampoo, then rinse. Towel off excess water. Apply conditioner. Let set for about a minute. Rinse and towel blot again.

2 While the hair is still damp, smooth a dime-sized amount of gel (rubbed into a film in the palms of the hands) over the surface of the hair. Pass it back and forth all over the hair, depositing it on the ends and hair shaft, avoiding the scalp. Use more only if your damp hair soaks it up. (If gel is too sticky for you, try some customized "gelicone.")

3 Allow hair to air dry. (If you want it to dry quickly, use blow dryer with diffuser in place, passing over the head evenly.)

4 When hair is completely dry, you can take a bit more gel to separate and define sections of the hair.

A. J.'s hair is quintessential nineties, but its "roots" can be traced through the following classic men's short hairstyles, all of which (in some version) are still seen today.

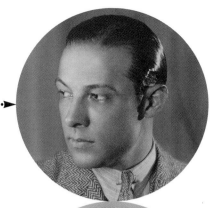

the city slicker—
neatly parted and combed flat against the head. The shine was integral to the look, accomplished with gobs and gobs of pomade. The epitome of the urban sophisticate, "man-after-dark" look even to this day.

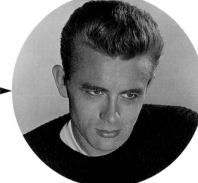

the rebel—
still seen today, this style progressed through the fifties through the nineties to become the forerunner of A. J.'s cut (with a little bit of loosening up). Back then, higher versions became known as "pompadours"; some had volumes of hair in back, fashioned into a "D.A." ("duck's ass"). Worn with or without a part, it needed lots of support at the roots, especially in front.

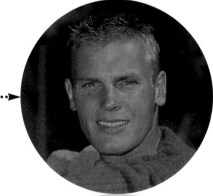

the serviceman—
the "buzz" or crew-cut was designed specifically with hygiene and grooming in mind. Kept this short, hair was less prone to poor health and did not require any styling time whatsoever. Truly the first wash-and-wear style. Has become the hallmark of hypermasculine good looks.

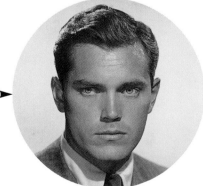

the collegiate—
"clean cut," parted on the side and held in place with a little Brylcreem or pomade, but not enough to make it appear too wet. This perennial "ivy-league" look has endured with little or no variation since the beginning of the century and is as popular today for the upwardly mobile male professional as it ever was.

For photo credits, see page 140.

A. J. Hammer, photographed by Don Flood

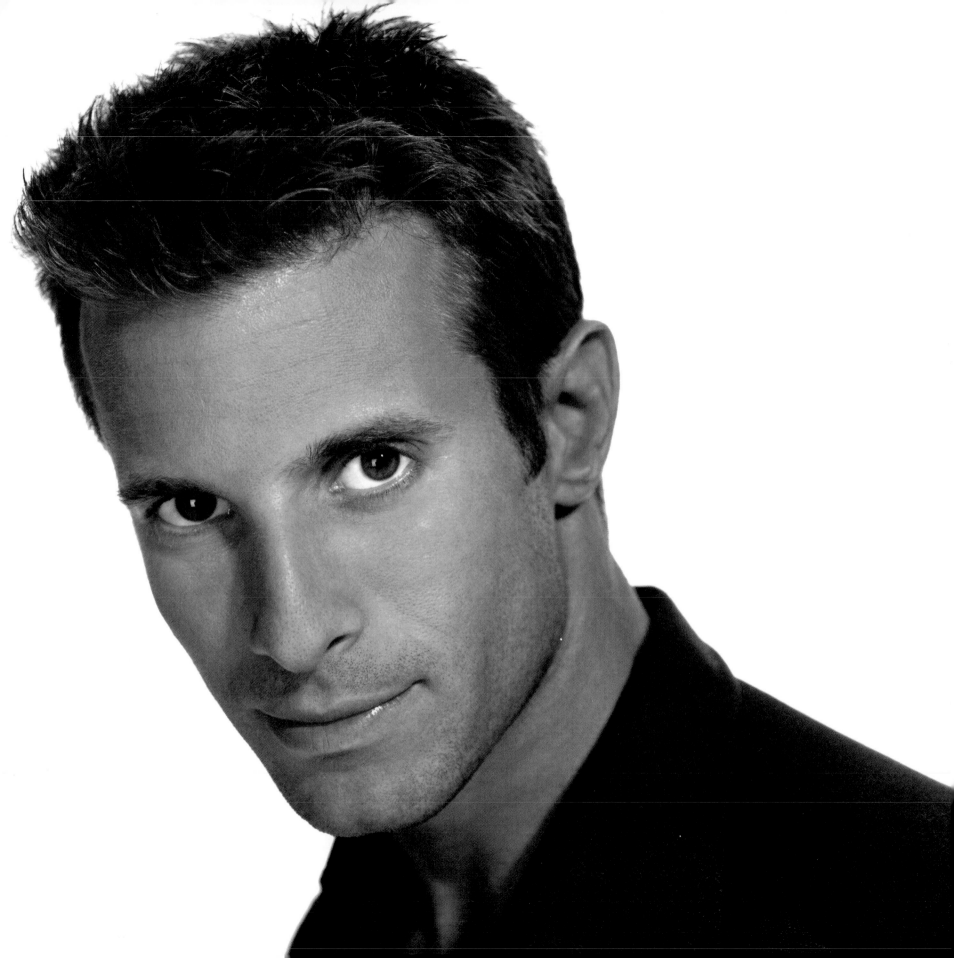

pomp
rigid roots to midshaft; soft, flexible ends, sides, and back

My good friend "Duff's" hair is usually worn down, in a signature free-swinging bob. However, on this occasion, styling her hair up and away from her face slightly elongates it and her normally pretty and tomboyish looks are transformed into something a bit more sophisticated.

1 Shampoo, rinse, and towel blot. Apply conditioner, comb through, and leave on for one to five minutes (depending on hair needs). Rinse, towel blot, and detangle hair with comb.

2 Concentrate volumizing spray into roots and along the length of top hairs, and a bit on the sides. Apply a small amount of creme groom (about a half-dime's worth) lightly to the sides and back of the hair.

3 With your dryer (with compression nozzle in place) and blow-drying brush, direct medium heat along the sides and back in a back-and-forth motion (to neutralize normal hair growth patterns and take out volume).

4 Once sides and back are flat and smooth to the head, move to the back of the top of the head. Using the same brush and dryer, lift hair straight up at the roots and apply hot air. Do in sections up to front hairline, working the hair up and back.

5 Using the round brush, smooth and polish top hair in sections (approximately five); heat hair while wrapped around brush, continually turning and polishing. While hair is still warm, immediately curl each section around rollers, directing the hair toward the back.

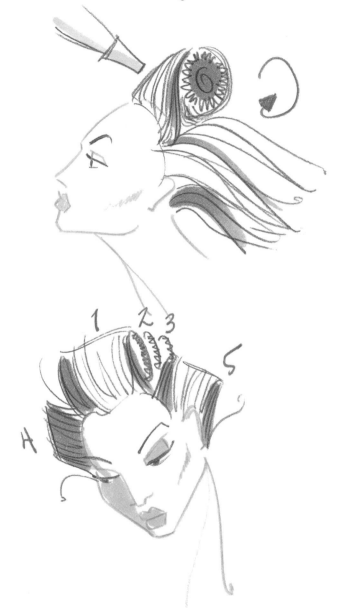

6 Spray rolled hair lightly with holding spray. Allow to cool and set. Remove rollers and massage in a very small amount of creme groom, using a backward motion.

7 Use comb to lift and shape style into place, lightly spraying as you move along. Spritz overall shape when completed.

Karen Duffy, photographed by Nicolai Grosell

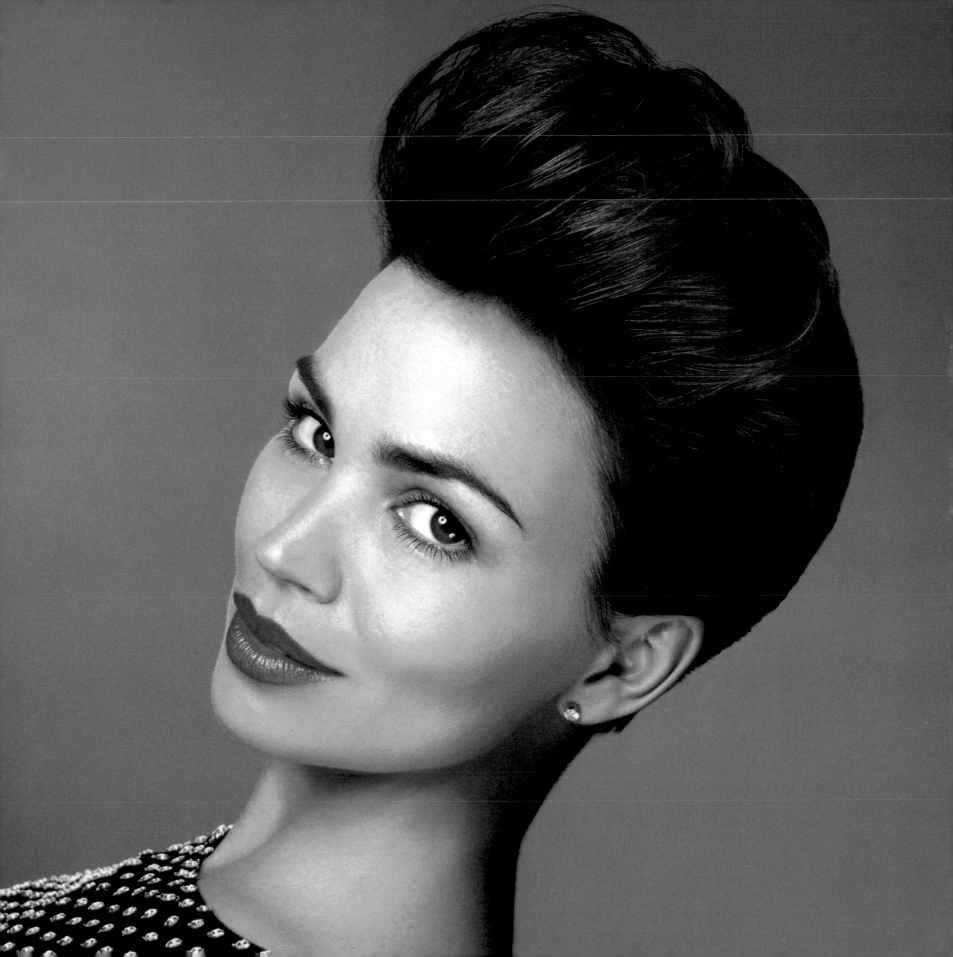

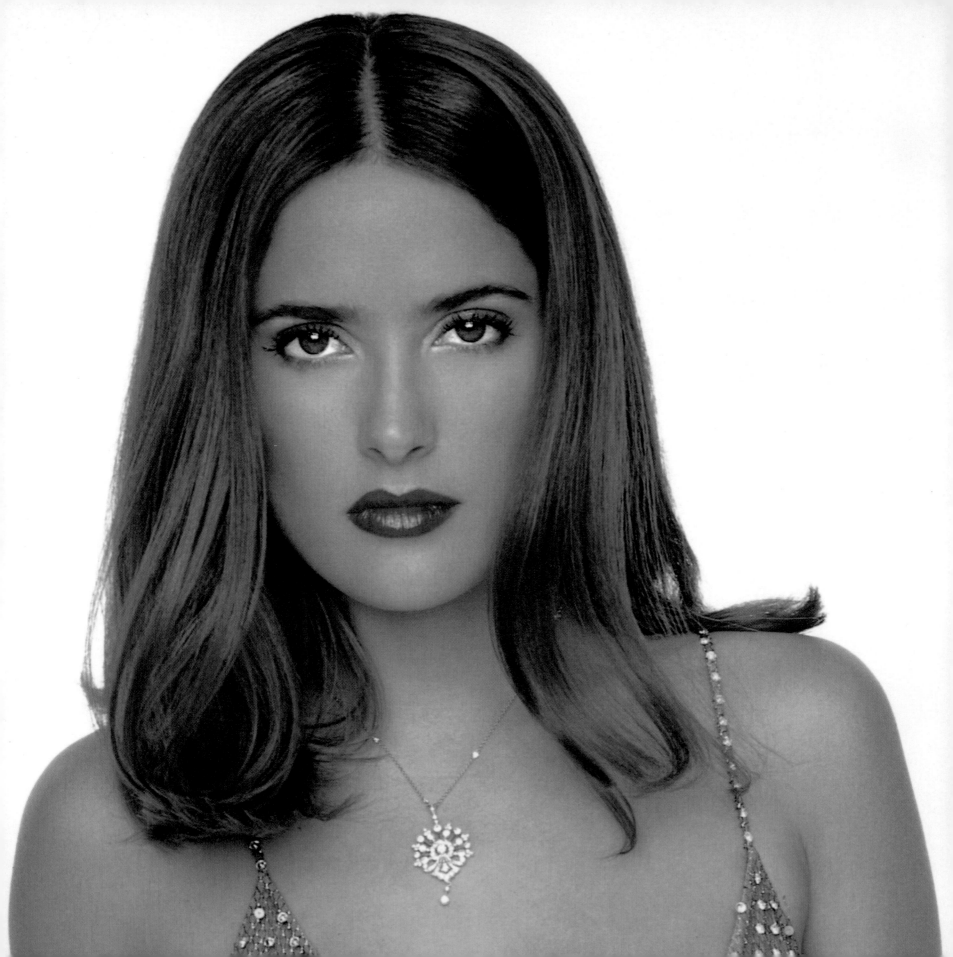

salma

hair type: thick and curly
special process: none
cut: simple one length with layers around face

tools

large-tooth comb • blow-drying brush
blow dryer with compressor • (large) round brush
flat iron (optional)

products

shampoo (for dry hair)
softening conditioner • straightening gel • silicone

Salma Hayek has fast become one of the most beautiful and talented new stars of the last few years. No doubt she can attribute part of her rise to fame to a very modern sense of style combined with just a touch of old Hollywood glamour. Gorgeous!

1 Shampoo, rinse, towel blot. Apply conditioner, comb through from roots to ends, and leave on for one to five minutes (depending on hair needs). Rinse and towel blot, removing all excess moisture. (You can even do a quick once-over with dryer.)

2 Smooth a thin layer of straightening gel on damp hair, from roots to ends, combing through. (Gel will also help detangle.)

3 Section hair from ear to ear across the back, and pin top portion to top of head.

4 For bottom layer of hair, set dryer (with compression nozzle in place) on high heat and use the blow-drying brush to pull down and straighten hair. Continue around to front hairline. Then release top hair section and repeat. When hair is dry, smooth a half-dime-size amount of silicone onto the hair. Then, with your round brush, smooth and polish hair to a lustrous shine.

Optional: For this picture, since Salma's hair is actually normally curly, I finished with a flat iron (starting at midshaft) to give it an even more naturally straight-textured look. However, I also gently curved the iron around the hair at the ends to give it subtle movement.

some famed long looks from the past:

Veronica Lake was the epitome of forties glamour, but her signature "peek a boo" hairstyle (draped seductively over one eye) was frowned upon in the workplace—it caused too many accidents owing to poor vision.

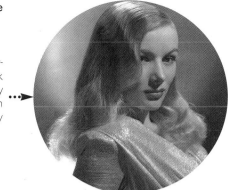

Typical (as if anything about Elizabeth Taylor could be) of the fifties was this pseudo-longish hairstyle that would just brush the shoulders. Incidentally, perming techniques had become relatively commonplace, so if you had straight hair putting in a wave or curl was an absolute necessity.

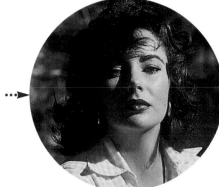

Were it not for the sixties, Cher, and her modish long, straight, jet black hair, where would we all be today? Everything about her haircut, from the length of the bangs to the brilliant simplicity of the sidepieces trimmed to accentuate the cheekbones, came together to create a true modern classic.

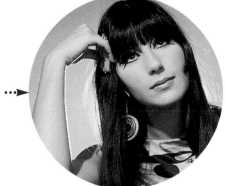

As fast as they change, many things remain the same. That's the case with the infamous Farrah Fawcett "shag." More an evolution than revolution in style, this look appealed as much to men because of its ultrafeminine charm as it did to women for the same reason, and has stayed with us in one modification or another (Jennifer Aniston's recent famed cut is a close cousin) for the past twenty-five or more years.

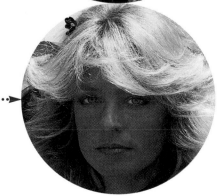

For photo credits, see page 140.

Salma Hayek, photographed by George Holz

hip
rigid roots to midshaft; flexible ends

rachel

hair type: straight, normal thickness
special process: brown highlights to "break up" denseness of natural color
cut: long layers, with soft long bangs and layers around face

tools
large-tooth comb • blow-drying brush
blow dryer with compressor • (large) round brush
large self-sticking rollers • paddle brush

products
shampoo (for color-treated hair) • reconstructing conditioner
volumizing spray • silicone • holding spray

Many women with straight black hair can feel somewhat limited in their styling choices. Typically, the idea of curling or double processing their hair for the sake of some variety seems like too much effort. And who can blame them for feeling this way, since straight hair textures are very difficult to manipulate? However, here the random highlighting of stunning actress Rachel Shane's hair to create the illusion of movement is a great example of a not-too-drastic process that can give you amazing results.

1 Shampoo, rinse, towel blot. Apply conditioner, comb through from roots to ends, leave on for one to five minutes (depending on hair needs). Rinse and towel blot.

2 On damp hair, spray volumizer all over, concentrating on root area at the top of the head. Add a touch of silicone to the ends.

3 Section hair from ear to ear across the back, and clip top section to top of head.

4 Using a blow dryer on high heat and blow-drying brush, blow hair straight while lifting at the roots. At the ends, switch to round brush for smoothing. Do this section by section until you reach the top of the head. Then use the blow-drying brush to lift at the roots, following with a round brush for more volume.

5 Simultaneously as you dry each top section, roll warm hair into self-sticking rollers, all the way to front hairline. Roll bang hair forward. Let cool.

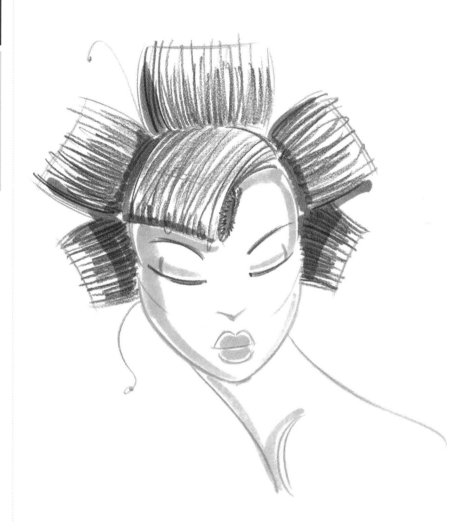

6 Remove rollers and brush with paddle brush in direction shown in photo. (If hair needs any "redirection," do so at the roots first, using the blow-drying brush.)

7 Spritz with a touch of holding spray.

Note: The ends of Rachel's hair were thinned to decrease its density, which would normally not allow it to be styled this "weightlessly." Additionally, for this photo, a little back combing was done on top for added height.

Rachel Shane, photographed by Nicolai Grosell

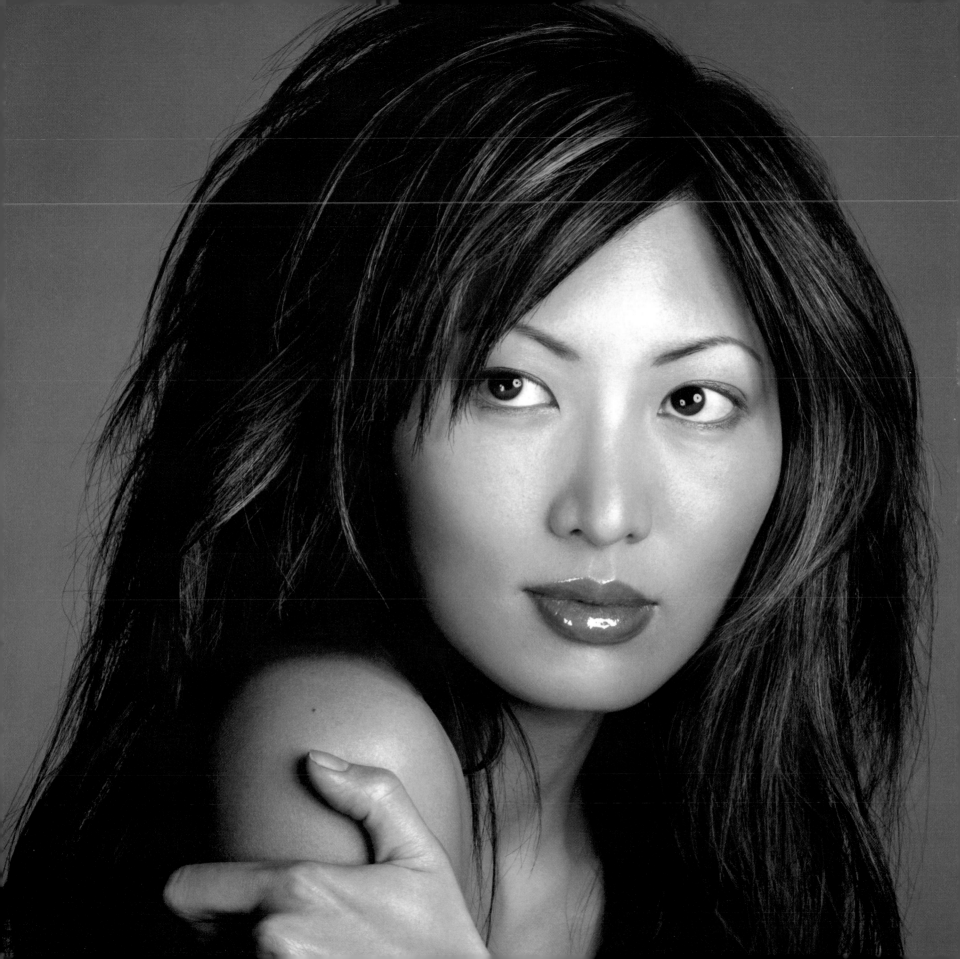

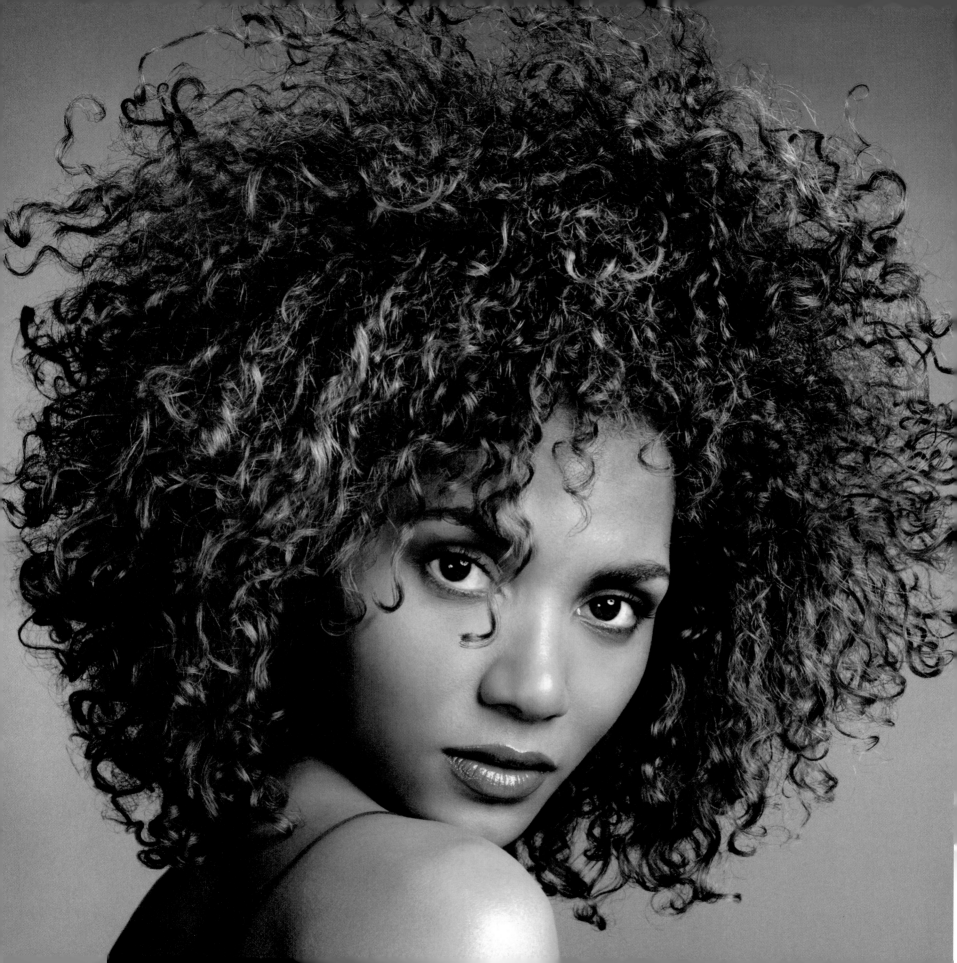

halle

hair type: medium soft, curly-kinky
special process: mild relaxing; golden auburn brown coloring
cut: round, layered

tools
large-tooth comb • tail comb • fork pick

products
shampoo and reconstructing conditioner (for color-treated hair)
leave-in conditioner • spray silicone

I never want to oversimplify things, but as you can see, there are only four steps to this wonderful freestyle look. But if your hair starts out as beautiful and naturally curly as lovely Halle Berry's, you'll see that very little effort is involved in accomplishing such a showstopper. By the way, this is one of those "hair supported by hair" styles that is possible because of the curly-kinky texture.

1 Shampoo, rinse, towel blot. Apply reconstructing conditioner, comb through to detangle, leave on for one to five minutes (depending on hair needs). Rinse and shake hair to remove excess water.

2 Add leave-in conditioner, squeezing it in (do not use comb or you will lose the curl). Rinse, leaving a bit of conditioner in hair. Shake again to remove excess water and let dry. (You may want to keep a towel around your shoulders to catch any dripping water.)

3 As your hair is drying, squeeze the curls gently, adding a touch of silicone.

4 When hair is completely air dried, lightly spritz on more silicone (for shine and definition) and separate curls, using tail of a tail comb, into looser, smaller pieces. Use the fork pick at the roots to lift and separate hair into support base. This is a style best achieved with a good eye for balance. Note: Always remember to choose the weight of a product (such as spray silicone, which is a very light formulation) and amount of product you use by the condition and quality of hair you're defining. Don't weigh it down.

Marcelled waves and pin curls
In the twenties, it was all the rage to have your hair marcelled (named for the man who perfected the technique) or finger waved. This was a perming procedure done very close to the scalp in an undulating pattern. Often it would be accentuated with pin curls (sometimes spit curls) placed along the hairline. The hair was kept in place while drying with pins and often lacquered with pomades. A great classic look shown here on Josephine Baker.

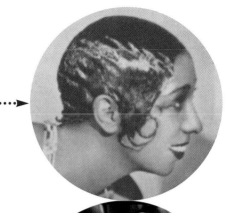

Corkscrews and cascading curls
During the forties, even if a woman's hair wasn't downright curly, you could be sure there would be plenty of wave in it. Beautiful Rita Hayworth had naturally dense and curly hair that would alternate between loose corkscrews (as seen here) and glamourous cascading waves. Her image during the period, seen in countless films and photos, became an ideal for women all over the world.

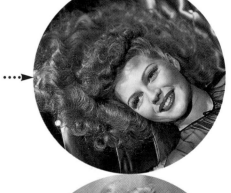

Goldilocks
There has never been a more famous child star than Shirley Temple, and probably never will be again. She owed much of her success to adorable, cherubic looks. So much so that mothers worldwide used her as a standard when dressing and grooming their own children. Her mother took time out every evening to set in place the exact same number of curls atop her head—fifty-six.

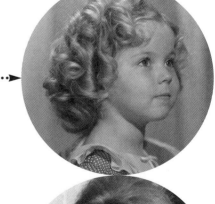

Tendrils
These curly wisps of hair are named for the parts of a plant, like a vine, that splinter off and spiral their way around an object. With hair, they add an immediate yet subtle touch of sexiness to the up styles they frequently accompany, and are either worn loose and free-floating or tightly curled. In the early sixties, Brigitte Bardot may have been solely responsible for bringing this casually elegant touch to women's hair.

For photo credits, see page 140.

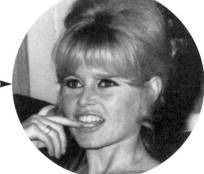

Halle Berry, photographed by Nicolai Grosell

sweep

niki

hair type: baby fine, wavy
special process: bleach highlights
cut: one-length back with angled layer front

tools

large-tooth comb • blow-drying brush
blow dryer with compressor • (medium) round brush
large U-shaped pins (or large bobby pins)
medium-barrel curling iron

products

shampoo and reconstructing conditioner (for fine, bleached hair)
lightweight softening conditioner (for detangling)
volumizing spray • clay groom • lightweight holding spray

I added just a couple of my own touches to this simple upswept hairstyle. Fabulous Niki Taylor was the perfect model in this portrait taken by the equally fab photog Sante D'Orazio.

1 Shampoo, rinse, towel blot.

2 Apply reconstructing conditioner and comb through, leave on for one to five minutes, rinse. Apply softening conditioner to ends only, rinse, and towel dry. (Deep condition twice a week.)

3 Spray hair all over with volumizing spray.

4 Turn head over, dry hair with dryer (on high heat) and blow-drying brush, brushing in all directions.

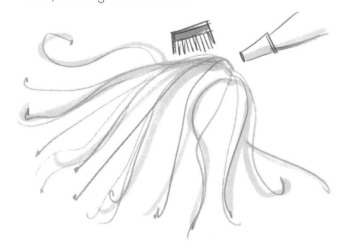

5 With head up, continue drying in same manner until hair is almost completely dry.

6 Using a round brush with the dryer, smooth and polish the hair, especially the ends and front.

7 Add clay groom to hair in sections, brush smooth and gather as if you were making a high ponytail (allowing pieces in front to drop out). Twist hair and roll into an *upside-down* version of the up-twist, tucking ends inside using U-shaped or bobby pins.

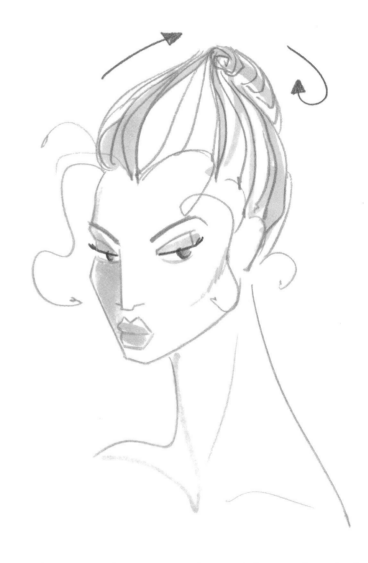

8 Use curling iron on loose pieces. Place with fingers about the head and spray lightly.

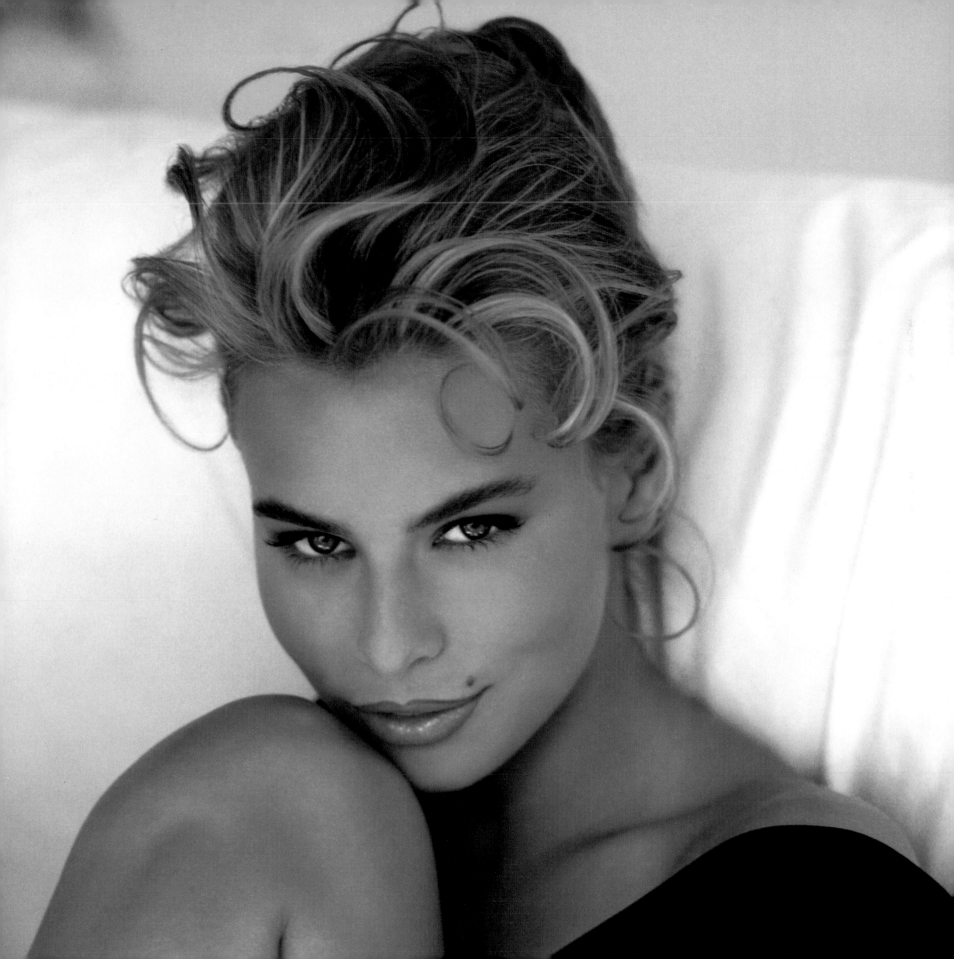

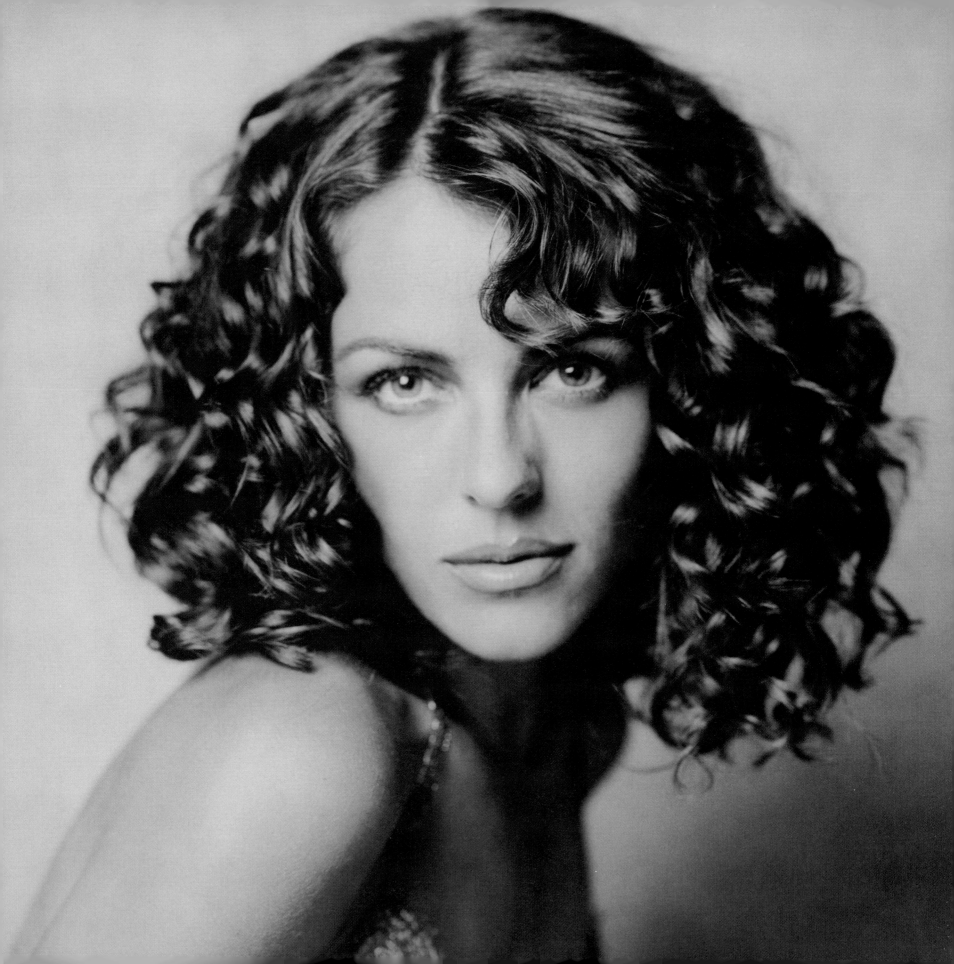

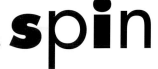

elizabeth

hair type: normal thickness, straight
special process: caramel brown highlights
cut: one-length back with angled layers front

tools

large comb with medium-spaced teeth • (medium) round brush
blow dryer with compressor • small-barrel curling iron

products

shampoo (for normal hair) • lightweight reconstructing conditioner
styling spray (or mousse) • silicone

I am fortunate to have worked with Elizabeth Hurley many times. This curly style is a departure for her; normally she sports straighter, albeit still glamorous looks. But Elizabeth is one of those rare beauties who can look good wearing any hairstyle.

1 Shampoo, rinse, towel blot.

2 Apply conditioner and comb through, leave on for one to five minutes, rinse; leave hair damp.

3 Apply styling spray (or mousse) to hair, adding a little extra to the roots for support, and comb through.

4 Section hair across back of head, from ear to ear, and pin to top of head.

5 Take a loose section and, using round brush, blow hair in an outward, rounding movement. Unclip and do the top. Do this until all hair is dry and ends are smooth.

6 Apply a thin film of silicone, especially on the ends.

7 Make a soft off-center part and split the hair into three sections, from side to side and across the back.

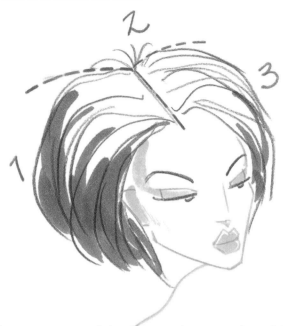

8 For curling, section small (approximately one inch wide) pieces of hair and wind around iron in a downward line from scalp. Hold clamp in place for a few seconds and gently release. Continue around head, piece by piece, section by section. Be careful with the hot iron. (As an alternate method, try using bendable sticks or small sponge rollers. Just remember to twist the individual hair sections first.)

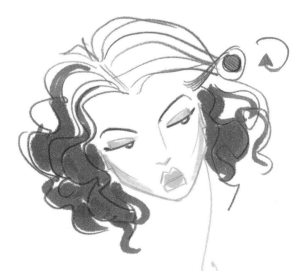

9 Finish by taking a light film of silicone to separate and define each curl (here I divided each into three smaller curls) with your fingertips. Be gentle and try not to overseparate curls, creating too much volume.

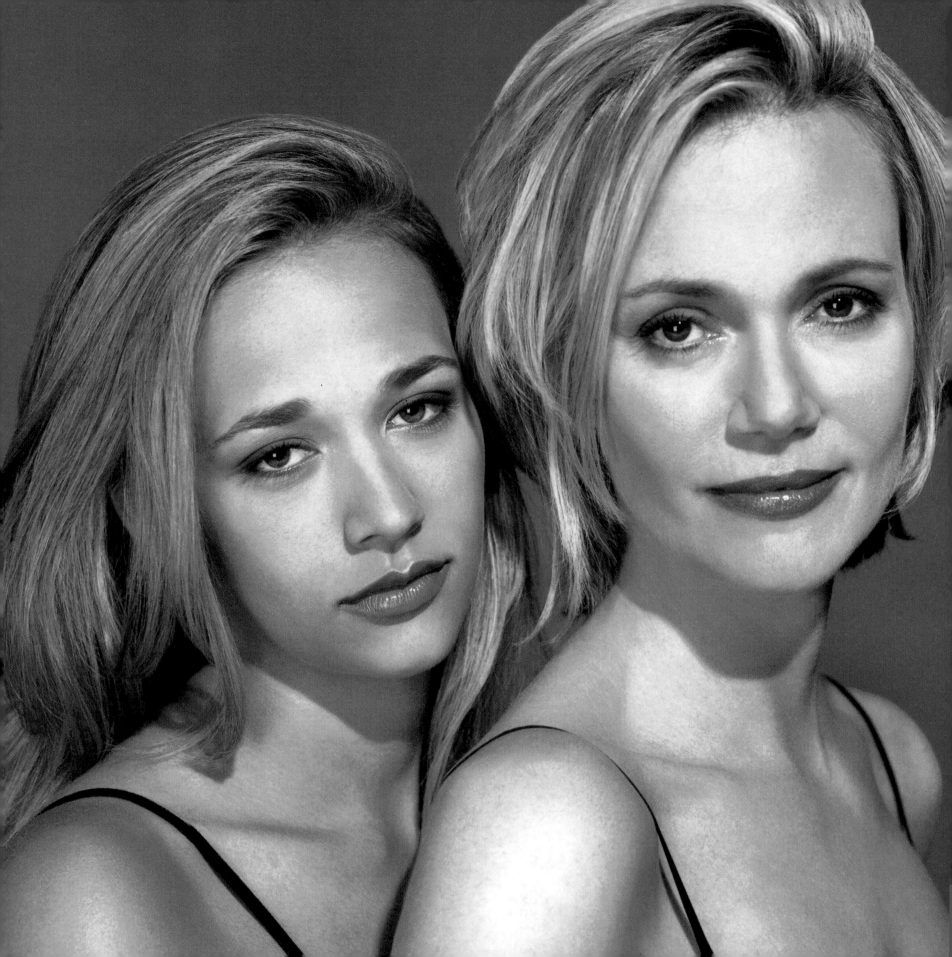

trio

rashida: rigid roots; soft midshaft to ends
peggy: rigid roots to midshaft; flexible ends
kidada: soft and flexible from roots to ends

When arrangements were first being made to schedule Peggy Lipton for her portrait, the idea of including her daughters, Rashida and Kidada (by music impresario Quincy Jones), was discussed. I had to think for a moment (but just for a moment). I knew Peggy was quite beautiful, but only fleetingly remembered seeing pictures of her children. But it immediately dawned on me what a golden opportunity I would have to show how hair texture can vary among family members, retaining its own beautiful individuality. I think you'll have to admit, looking at this picture, that I couldn't illustrate the point better than with these three gorgeous subjects.

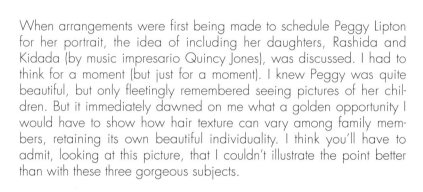

Rashida Jones, Peggy Lipton, and Kidada Jones, photographed by Don Flood

rashida

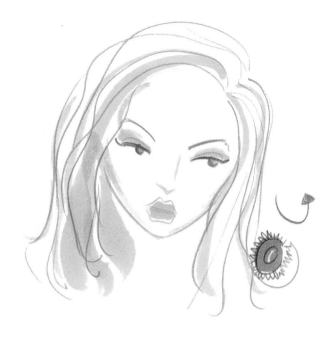

hair type: baby fine, curly to wavy
special process: foil highlights with a pale ash tint
cut: long layers with angled front

tools
large-tooth comb • blow dryer with compressor and diffuser
(medium to small) round brush • finishing brush

products
shampoo (for baby-fine hair)
reconstructing conditioner (for color-treated hair)
softening conditioner (for detangling)
silicone • volumizer spray
styling spray • clay groom

1 Shampoo, rinse, towel blot.

2 Comb reconstructing conditioner through hair, leave for a few moments, rinse, and blot.

3 Apply softening conditioner to hair from midpoint to the ends and comb through, rinse, and towel blot.

4 Smooth small amount of silicone on hair for more detangling. Use volumizer spray at roots on top of head. Use styling spray over remaining hair and ends.

5 With diffuser in place, pass dryer over hair with head turned upside down. Squeeze in wave using fingers. Also use fingertips to rub root area to create more volume. Dry roots completely, but leave rest of hair damp.

6 When you turn your head right side up it will look pretty wild. We don't want to lose the fullness, but we want to tame and shape it around the front hairline and ends.

7 Roll a manageable amount of hair around the round brush and apply heat from the dryer (with compression nozzle in place) to smooth, polish, and refine. Do this all over, creating flips and turns in the hair and maintaining lift at the top. Cool each section as you go along.

8 Brush through with finishing brush. Then, with a small amount of clay groom, smooth and separate hair to give it the look of more movement. If you like, finish with a touch of styling spray.

peggy

hair type: normal thickness, smooth and straight with body
special process: bleach and tint highlights with a golden tone
cut: nonprecision shaglike shape with choppy, spiked layering

tools
foundation brush • blow dryer with compressor
(medium) round brush • straightening tongs
hard rubber comb (optional)

products
shampoo (for color-treated hair) • softening conditioner
reconstructing conditioner • volumizing spray
silicone • clay groom

1 Shampoo, rinse, towel blot.

2 Apply softening conditioner, rinse, towel blot. (Normally, for this type hair, apply reconstructing conditioner twice a week.)

3 Spray volumizer to roots at crown and lightly overall on the ends.

4 Gather all hair together and smooth a bit of silicone just on the ends.

5 Section hair from ear to ear across back and fasten to top of head.

6 Using foundation brush and dryer, blow hair down, not out, and rounded.

7 Continue drying this way until you reach the natural curve of the head. Switch to a round brush and dry hair while pulling it away from the scalp for volume.

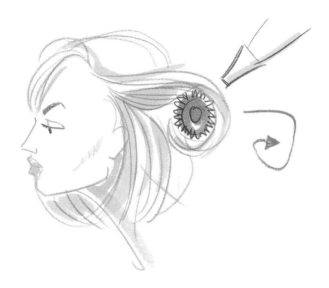

8 At the bang and part area, blow and dry hair up and back to create lift.

9 When hair is completely dry, smooth with straightening tongs to reduce any extra volume. (You can also use the hard rubber comb with a dryer to get rid of any unwanted roundness or volume.)

10 Rub about a half dime's worth of clay groom into the palms of your hands and work into the hair section by section. Then separate hair into chunky bits.

kidada

hair type: tight curl and kink, medium thickness
special process: relaxed, highlighted with reddish brown tints
cut: simple, straight, one-length to chin with jagged edges

tools
blow-drying brush • blow dryer with compressor
(medium) round brush •

products
shampoo (for dry or color-treated hair) • reconstructing conditioner
softening conditioner • straightening gel
silicone • clay groom

1 Shampoo, rinse, towel blot. Apply reconstructing conditioner, set for five minutes, rinse, blot, apply softening conditioner, rinse, and blot. (Alternate method: Apply reconstructor to ends while hair is dry, wet and shampoo hair, concentrating on cleansing roots. Rinse, and comb through softening conditioner, concentrating on shaft and ends. Rinse. This method is especially good for anyone with extralong hair or hair with mixed textures and different needs.)

2 Smooth straightening gel over hair, concentrating on ends (and tough, frizzy spots like those around the hairline).

3 Section hair from ear to ear along back and pin to top of head. Using dryer and blow-drying brush, straighten hair. (Always pull hair downward and follow brush with immediate stream of high-heat airflow, switching to cool as hair dries.)

4 When this section is dry, use medium round brush and dryer to smooth ends. (If necessary, a small application of silicone can be added if hair is very dry.)

5 Continue drying top part of head, creating a smooth scalp shape and defined "zigzag" part (see page 37) by blowing the hair straight down and flat at the part area.

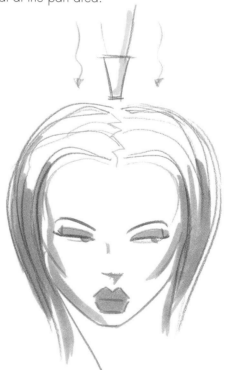

6 Use a bit of clay groom to smooth flyaways and give hair shine and pliability.

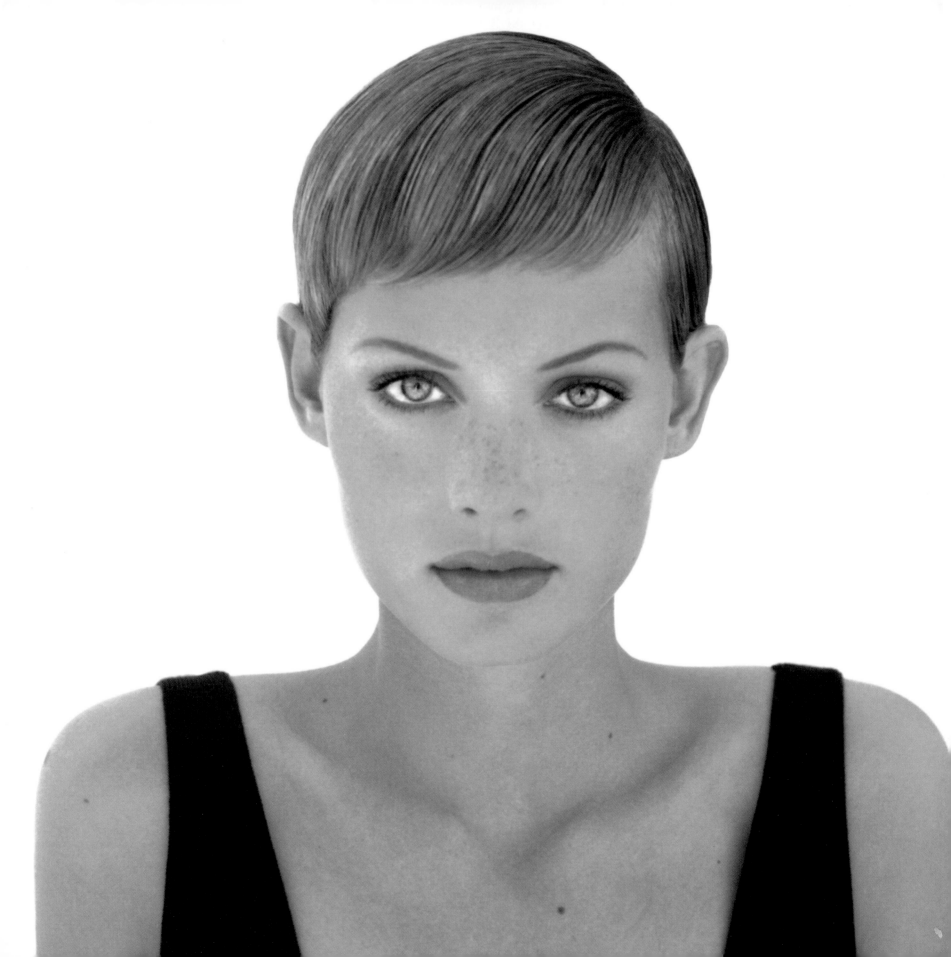

amber

hair type: curly, medium coarse
special process: none
cut: short bowl shape, razored around edges, bangs softened with thinning shears

I chose to include this picture for one major reason: to illustrate the simple beauty of a great cut. Basically, Amber jumped into the pool and came out looking more or less like this. All I did was comb the hair into one direction and smooth the bangs in place with my finger. If you want to see what her hair looks like without the combing, check out the miniature reprint of the cover of *Harper's Bazaar* on page 13.

Beginning with a great cut, a style like this can easily be achieved with the application of your own custom-blended product: in this case, mixing gel and silicone to get "gelicone" for a wet *and* soft look. Just shampoo, condition, and rinse normally. While hair is still damp, apply "gelicone" and comb into place using a medium-tooth comb. Then, using the edge of the comb or fingers, direct the bangs to the desired side.

short 'n' sweet

While great cuts are not limited to those worn short, a good number of them owe much of their success to their brevity. The four women opposite represent just a small sampling of the many classic diminutive 'dos from over the years.

Louise Brooks—
Before the 1920s, women were expected to keep their hair long, although, oddly enough, never down (unless they were in the bedroom). Though Brooks was not the first to "bob" her hair, her cut, deliberately shaped to accentuate her cheekbones, temples, and eyes, caused a sensation and was mimicked by women the world over.

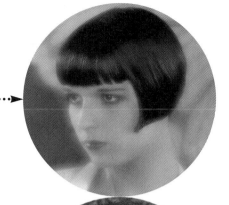

Audrey Hepburn—
This is a sort of trompe l'oeil hairstyle, meant to look short when in reality all the length was tucked away in back. During the 1950s, Hepburn excelled in this take on the "pixie-gamine," in direct opposition to her full-haired (and -bodied) peers, from Mansfield to Monroe. Hepburn did actually shed the extra hair in the early sixties, in a short cut that was trimmed to fit along the sides and lifted a bit at the crown for a touch of height.

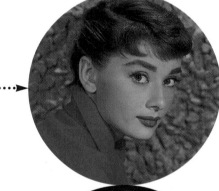

Mia Farrow—
Even though Jean Seberg did it in the late fifities (for "Saint Joan") and Twiggy became *the* sixties model because of it, it wouldn't be until Mia went from superlong to supershort that such a clipped cut would garner so much worldwide attention. At the time, she wanted off her very popular tv show "Peyton Place" and this single act became the perfect way to signal her frustration.

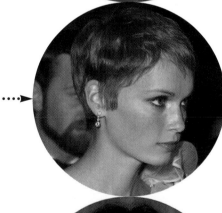

Dorothy Hamill— .
The two top haircuts of the seventies had to be Farrah Fawcett's "shag" and this Olympic medal winner's signature bob. Whether intentionally or not, her hair was left just long enough to exaggerate movement (such as the famous Hamill camel) without accidentally getting in the way of a flawless performance. Here truly form follows function.

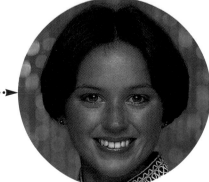

For photo credits, see page 140.

Amber Valetta, photographed by Patrick Demarchelier for Harper's Bazaar

cascade soft from roots to ends

brooke

hair type: mixed wavy and curly, coarse
special process: golden blond tinted highlights
cut: simple one length, angled front

tools
blow-drying brush • blow dryer with diffuser
medium-barrel curling iron

products
shampoo (for dry coarse hair)
conditioner (for dry, chemically treated hair)
softening conditioner (optional: for detangling)
creme groom • silicone

Brooke Shields, among other things, is famous for her long, flowing hair. On this occasion, a cover for *Rolling Stone*, only a slight deviation from her normal fantastic self was in order. Since the finished style, with all its twists, curls, and mixed textures, reminded me of rushing water, I thought the name "cascade" was more than apt. Incidentally, if you're beginning with straight hair, you can get all the variegated qualities here by curling all your hair first, then pull and twist randomly on different sections.

1 Shampoo, rinse, towel blot. Add conditioner, rinse, towel blot. (Then add softening conditioner, if necessary. Rinse and blot.)

2 Apply creme groom over all hair and brush through. Part hair in center.

3 Using dryer with diffuser (on high heat), twist and smooth hair in small sections, while gently pulling curl out. Do this until entire head is dry.

4 Use curling iron on random sections to create uneven pattern.

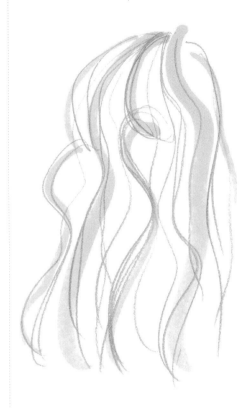

5 Add silicone to finish and define.

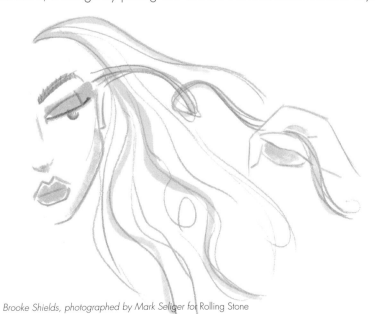

Brooke Shields, photographed by Mark Seliger for Rolling Stone

122

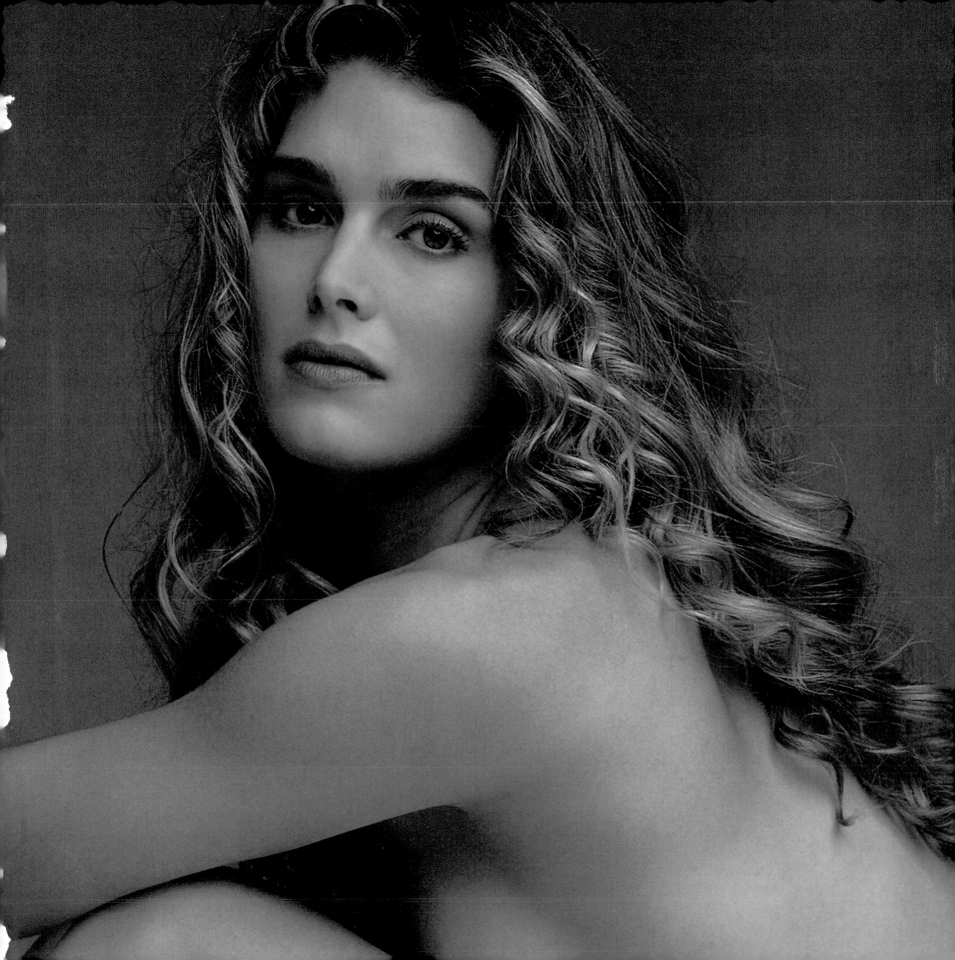

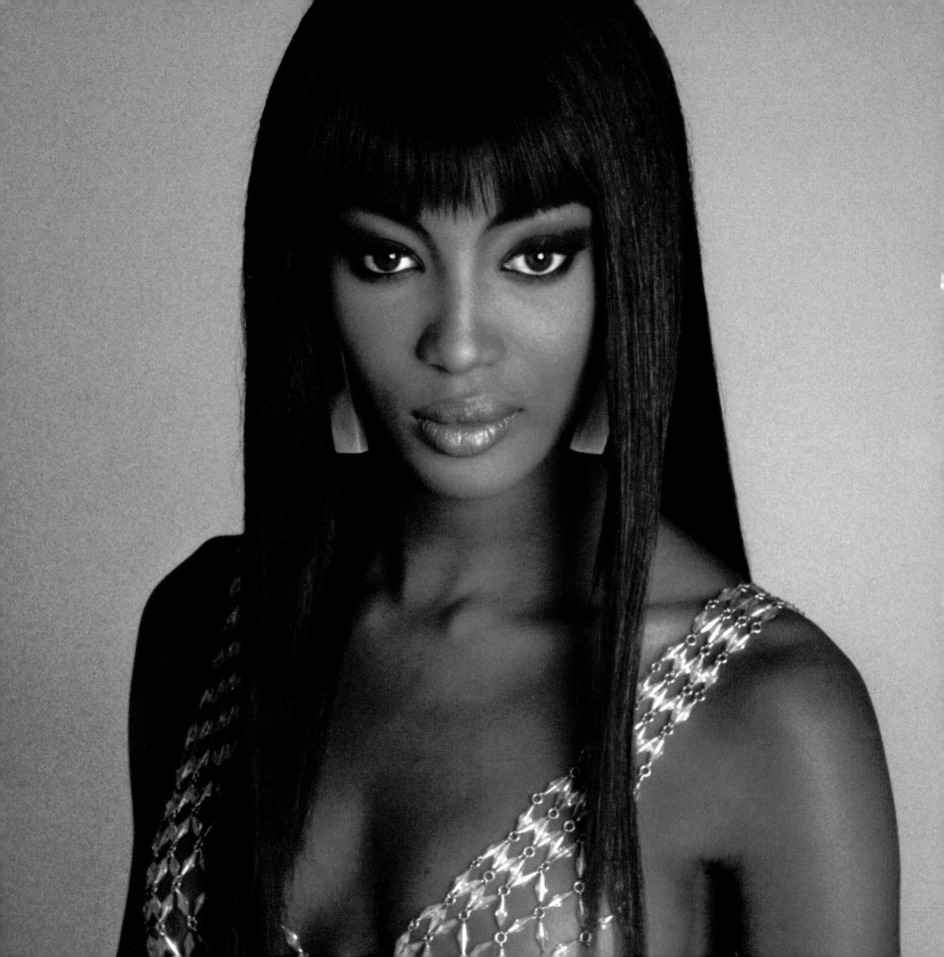

naomi

hair type: thick and curly
special process: light highlights with permanent color
cut: long layers with angled front

tools
fine-tooth comb • blow-drying brush
blow dryer with compressor • (large) round brush • flat iron

products
shampoo and conditioner (for relaxed hair)
straightening gel • silicone • holding spray

I have been a huge fan of Naomi Campbell's ever since she became a model a few years back. She almost singlehandedly changed the business, showing the world that fashion and beauty should have no color boundaries. But even beyond that, her extreme versatility and beauty have allowed individuals like myself to create an amazing range of looks on her, from drop-dead glamour (as seen here through the eyes of master photographer Francesco Scavullo), to casual sophistication (see an *Allure* cover of her in miniature on page 14).

Basically, the steps for this style are exactly the same as for Stephanie Seymour's "slide" on page 100 and Salma Hayk on page 107, with one exception. Since Naomi's hair was relaxed, I was particularly careful not to be overly aggressive when straightening it and did not add the extra bend to the ends.

Throughout this book, I have referred to many of the cuts pictured in terms of different levels of layering. As a way of further explaining the point, I have chosen a trio of illustrations to show the range of variations.

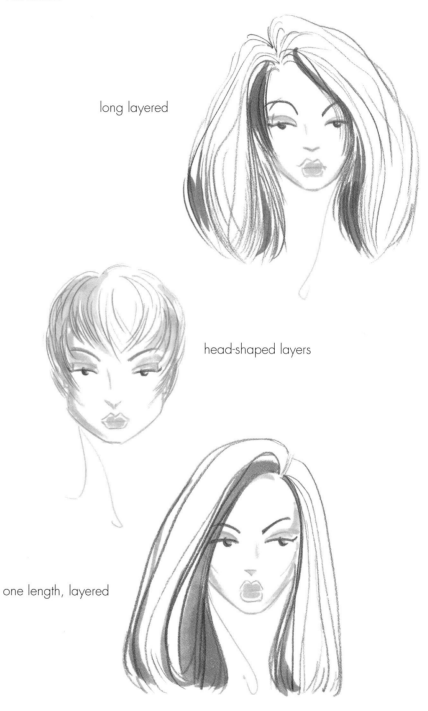

long layered

head-shaped layers

one length, layered

freestyle rigid roots; flexible ends

drew

hair type: thick and wavy
special process: pale, golden blond tints
cut: short and spiky with uneven layers made with razor and shears

tools
hard rubber comb • blow dryer with compressor or diffuser

products
shampoo and softening conditioner (for color-treated hair)
clay groom (or pomade)

This is one of those simple, simple styles/textures that's been a favorite look for quite some time now. It has a youthful, exuberant quality to it that brings out the "rebel" in whoever is wearing it. Delightful Drew Barrymore makes a great rabble-rouser.

1 Shampoo, rinse, and towel blot.

2 Apply conditioner, leave on for a few moments, rinse, and blot.

3 Rub a small amount of clay groom (about the size of a pea) into palms and apply to hair by pulling out individual sections. (You can use the corner tip of your comb to help separate chunks.) When you're done, your hair should look like a wet porcupine.

4 Using the dryer on low heat, blow your hair dry in all directions. Be careful not to blow apart hair that has been sectioned.

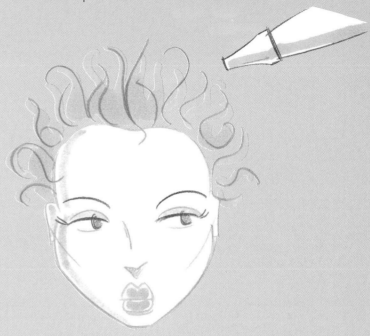

5 When it is completely dry, use a touch more groom to spike hair in all directions. Use the photo as a guide.

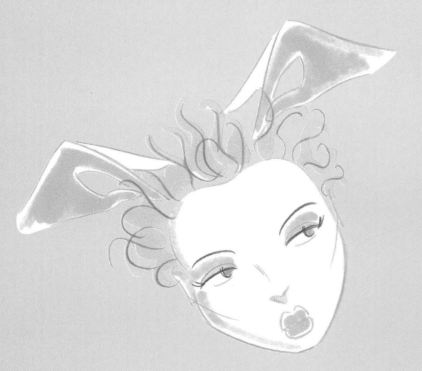

Drew Barrymore, photographed by Wayne Maser

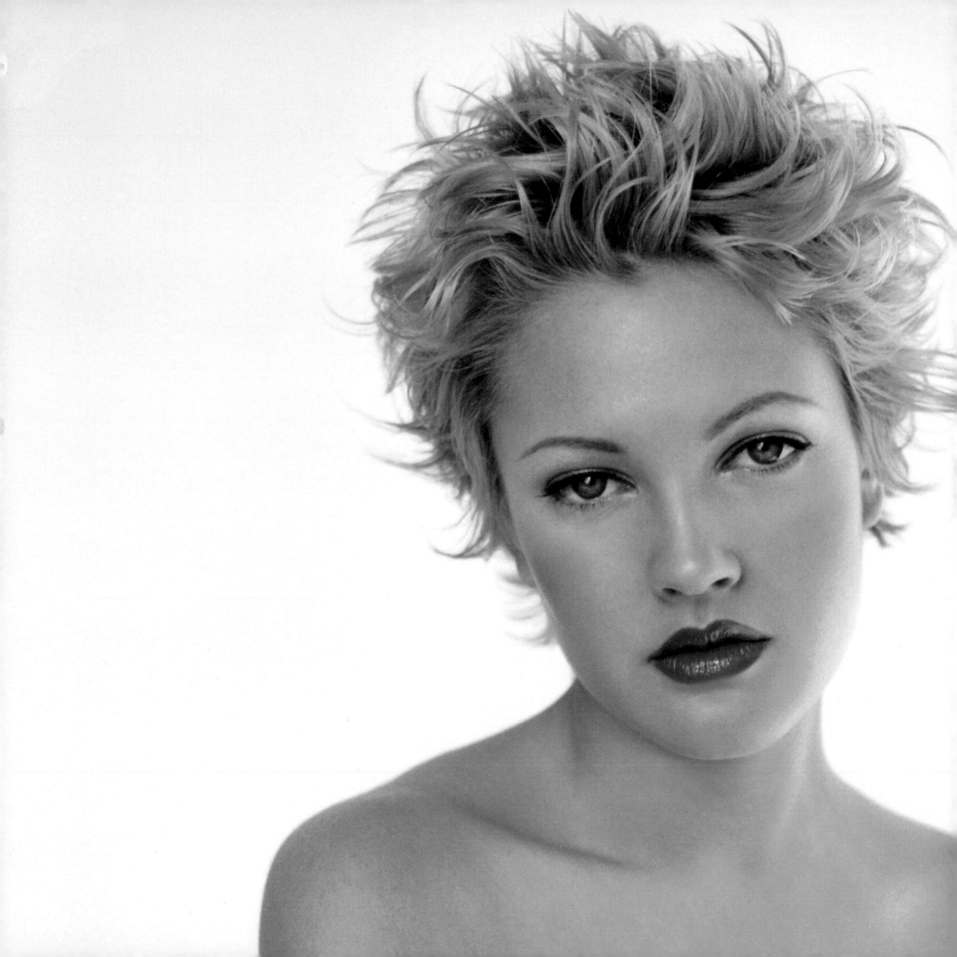

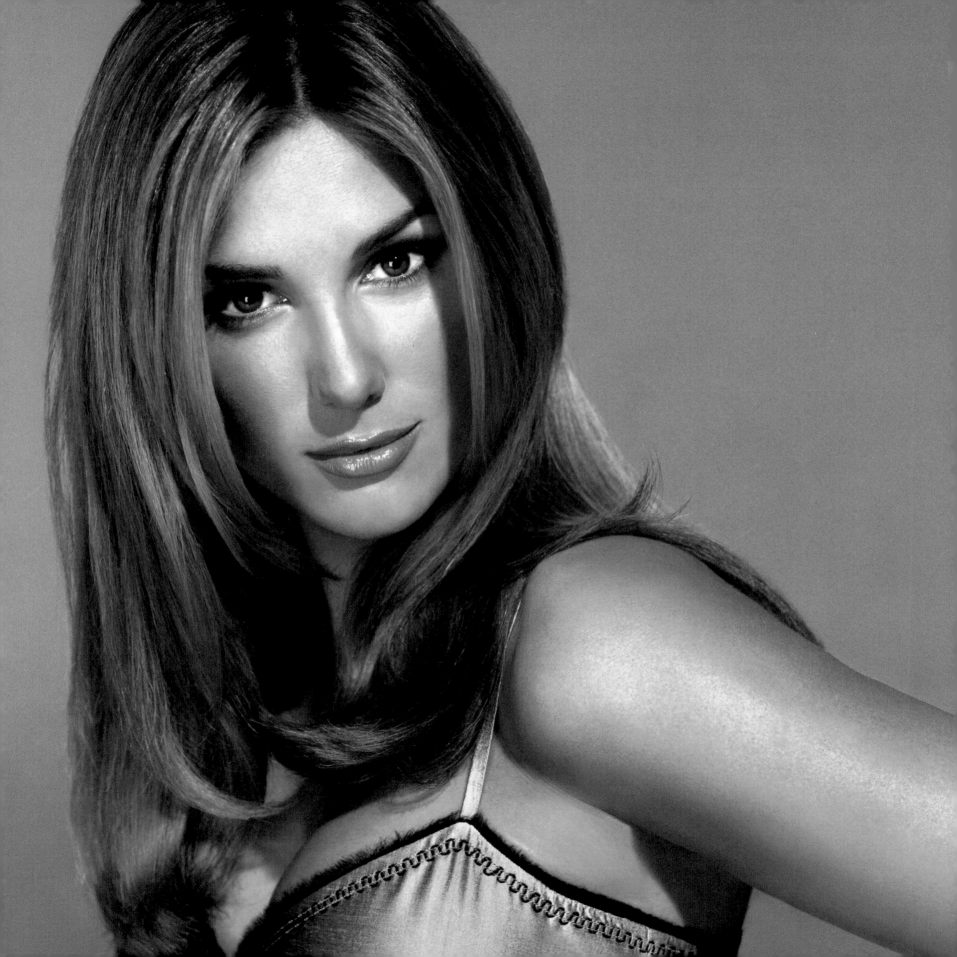

daisy

hair type: thick and curly
special process: light highlights with permanent color
cut: long layers with angled front

tools
medium-tooth comb • blow-drying brush
blow dryer with compressor • (large) round brush • paddle brush

products
shampoo and conditioner (for normal hair)
straightening gel • creme groom

Divine Daisy Fuentes has the kind of hair that, because of its beautiful natural texture, can look great from stick straight all the way to extremely curly. This tousled wave style is somewhere in between the two (leaning a bit closer to straight) and is very easy to do, especially once you've mastered the basic hair-straightening method. The look is modern, sexy, and flattering.

1 Shampoo, rinse, and towel blot. Apply conditioner with comb, wait, rinse, and blot again.

2 Apply a film of straightening gel evenly to damp hair.

3 Section hair across the back and pin on top.

4 Using your blow-drying brush and dryer, proceed to straighten the hair. When hair is almost dry, switch to the round brush and "polish" smooth. (Creme groom can be added to ends for more control). Continue up to front hairline.

5 Finish by applying a light film of creme groom all over hair (for fly-aways, etc.) and brush through with your paddle brush. Then just toss your head around and see what happens to the hair naturally.

the long and short of it

During the early part of the century, even though almost all women kept their hair long, it was always worn up. This was because long hair was considered too provocative to be worn down, especially in public. More telling, though, was the fact that it was considered a grave act of misconduct to cut it, even compelling some husbands to divorce wives who did. However, by the twenties, after the suffragette movement, women made a stand and the "bob" was born. Revolutionary as it was, it was only temporary. Places like Hollywood would do their best to equate long hair with glamour, femininity, and the evening, and short hair with matronliness, masculinity, and daytime—and they succeeded. It wouldn't be until the fifties that there was some overlap, so to speak, of lengths, but longish hair was still associated with femininity, although there was some room for the slightly tomboyish role of a gamine. Finally, by the sixties, women (and men, too) let their hair down once and for all. Thankfully, this newfound freedom to some degree vanquished the notion that women could be limited by their hairstyle. Today we are expected to believe that a woman can wear her hair at any length she chooses—she can clip it up, or leave it loose—and not be thought any more or less feminine, either way. Whether or not we have actually gotten past those old stereotypes remains to be seen. Although I can't speak for anyone else in this regard, I have never considered one option more or less attractive than the other. As far as hair is concerned, long or short, I only see the possibilities, not the limitations.

shorn soft

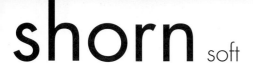

john

hair type: coarse, thick, and curly
special process: none
cut: barbered short

tools
brush

products
shampoo and conditioner (for normal hair)
styling gel or creme groom

Ask anyone how a guy looks his best, and I guarantee you they'll answer with one word: natural. The idea of a man trying *too* hard to look good just doesn't seem to work. Now that doesn't mean he shouldn't try to look his best, but going overboard in the dressing and grooming department somehow makes him seem a bit narcissistic or pretentious (not to mention a touch insecure). Interestingly, the same is not necessarily true for a woman. In John's case, in going for that "natural" look, he's had to contend with that almost universal problem for men: loss of hair. However, as you can see, John is no less handsome for the lack of some locks. In fact, he may be even more attractive. One reason may be that he refuses to make a point of it by trying to camouflage or cover it up.

For men who find themselves in similar circumstances, I recommend reading through these basics:

- *Always maintain clean hair and a clean scalp*. You'd be surprised at how much of hair loss can be attributed to clogged pores. However, this does not mean you should be overly aggressive in the shampoo department, either. Too much cleansing will dry out the hair, causing other problems. Just be regular and diligent about it.

- *Keep the addition of grooming products in check*. Obviously, with a small amount of hair you shouldn't need to use much gel and so on. However, when hair is very short, it's often difficult to get it to lie down flat. The truth is, it may need to grow out just to where its own weight will allow it to flatten. Adding more product won't necessarily be the solution. You'll end up getting much more on your scalp than is good for you.

- *Be cautious with chemical treatments*. Admittedly, a lot of men color their hair, though probably not to the degree that women do. When gray hairs appear, some men are quick to head for the "bottle." Two bits of advice: If you are going to color over gray, do it as soon as you can. Don't wait for the gray to become so obvious that coloring over it will look obvious. (Remember, often with the advent of gray hair there is a lightening of the skin. Sometimes the contrast between it and recently colored hair is too drastic). If your hair is already suffering from loss, chemical processes such as relaxing and coloring will further weaken the follicles. Even if this doesn't accelerate the loss, you will have to keep your hair as conditioned and hydrated as possible.

- *Exercise and general health*. In this day and age, more and more men (and women) are getting into better physical shape. That is certainly the case with John. However, one nasty by-product of strenuous exercise is perspiration. While sweating is a necessary bodily function, an accumulation of it in the hair can eventually hurt it. Sweat, as you should know, contains salts, and this does not mix with hair. It will dry it out. While I won't say that most men are lazy, there are those of you out there who will only rinse with water after a workout. Often this is not enough to rid your hair of salt deposits. While you don't want to overcleanse your hair, do not leave something in it (like salt) that will only hurt it. On that note, your general health can affect some types of hair loss, and a change in diet may restore some hair growth. But not all, because it is generally understood that hair loss is probably genetic. Check on your mother's side of the family and see what's going on with her father. If he's bald or headed there, chances are pretty good, so be prepared.

- *Hair replacements and restorers*. Unfortunately, for most men, while the incidence of hair loss is common, the availability of successful alternatives is not. Too often hairpieces, including weaves and plugs, neither look natural nor function adequately. Often the only one being fooled is the wearer. If you are willing to pay the price (and it can be quite hefty), hair that is surgically implanted seems to be the best solution in this area. And if you hadn't noticed, there are a lot of top male stars who have submitted. But they can afford it. In the area of hair restorers, there does seem to be some real progress, especially for the common man, but the magic potions only work for some, not all. And what many men do not realize is that these can only work on restoring hair in places where it is thinning, not in spots where the hair is completely gone. This is another situation where, if you plan on using it, don't wait too long. If your shiny pate is showing, it might be too late.

John Francis, photographed by Don Flood

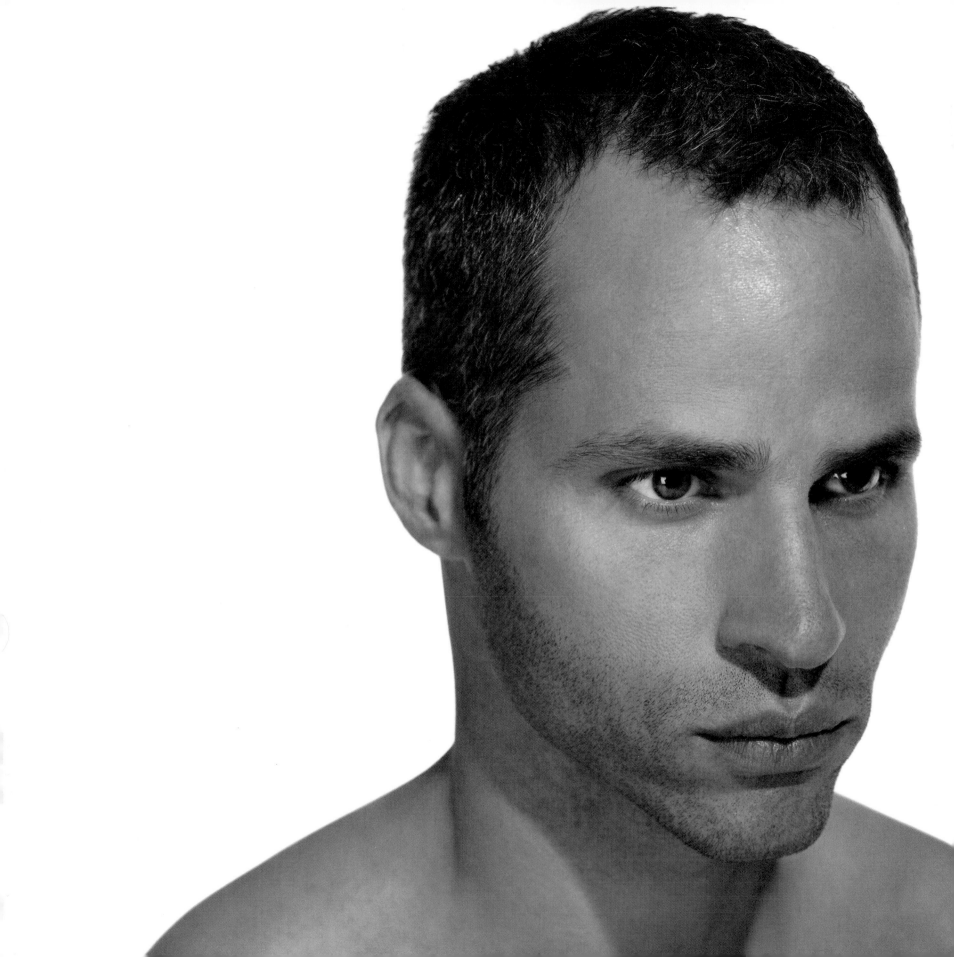

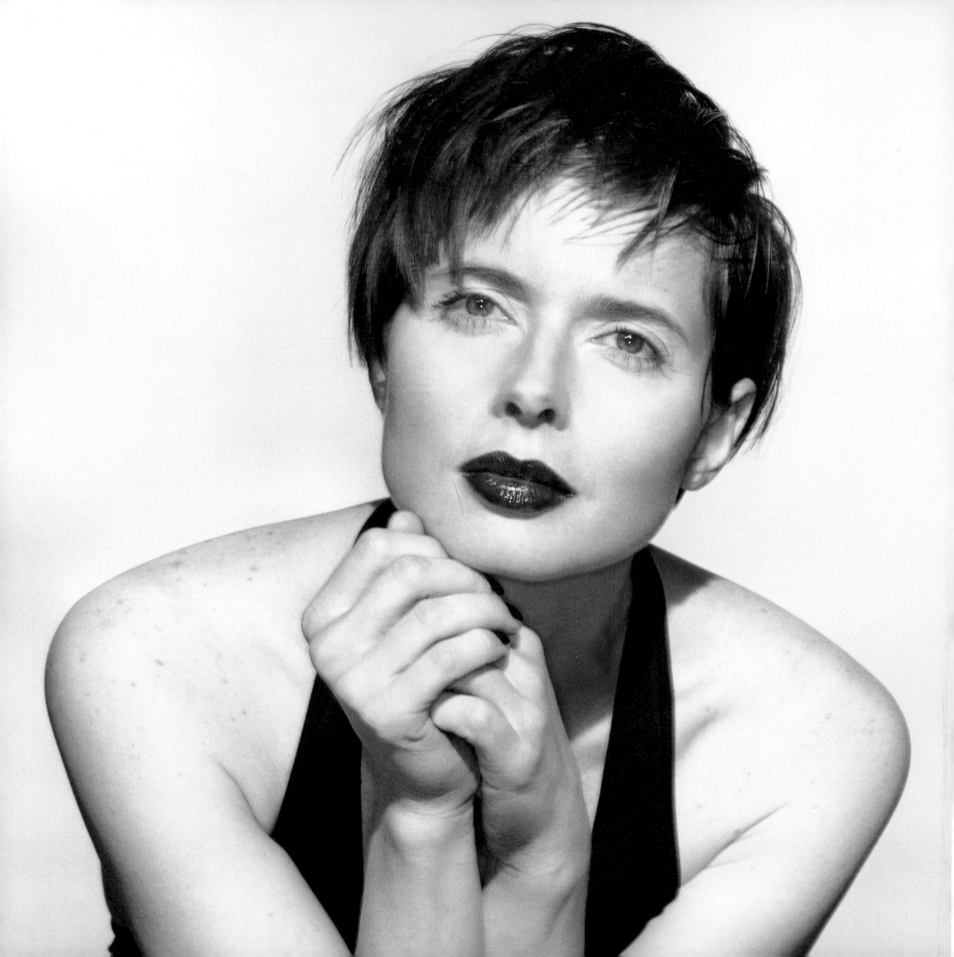

isabella

hair type: fine, straight
special process: color enhanced with brown tint
cut: razored and sheared short and layered

tools
blow-drying brush
blow dryer with compressor • (medium) round brush

products
shampoo and conditioner (for fine hair)
volumizing spray • clay groom

It's hard to imagine a person more gorgeous as Isabella Rossellini. As a modern day beauty icon she stands alone, and I believe not just for her superb looks, but because she is truly a nice person. Having worked with her often over the years, I have noticed her favoring shorter hair lengths, such as this one, but she still allows herself to remain visually versatile when the situation arises.

1 Shampoo, rinse, and towel blot.

2 Apply conditioner, leave for a few moments, rinse, and blot again.

3 Spray volumizer into root area and lightly on ends of hair.

4 Take blow dryer and brush and blow hair in all directions, adding extra lift at roots in crown area.

5 Apply a thin film of clay groom to hair in a "forward" direction.

6 Take the round brush and dryer and blow ends of hair toward face, twisting for a light curl.

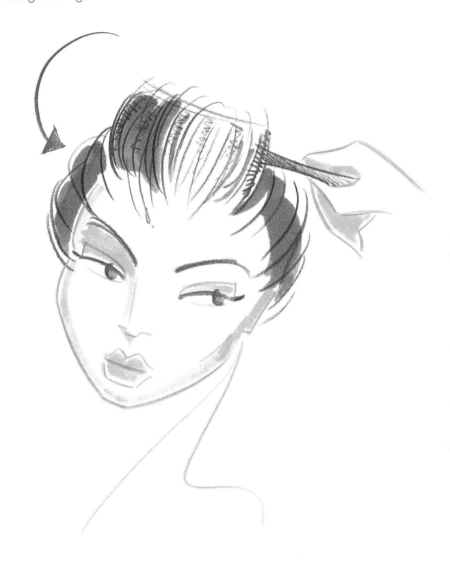

Isabella Rossellini, photographed by Gilles Bensimon

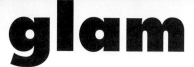

kristen

hair type: curly and thick
special process: permanent blond
cut: one-length back, angled front

tools

large-tooth comb • blow-drying brush
blow dryer with compressor • (large) round brush
large-barrel curling iron • styling clips
large self-sticking rollers (optional) • finishing brush

products

shampoo and softening conditioner (for color-treated hair)
reconstructing conditioner • straightening gel • styling spray
silicone • creme groom • holding spray

You would think playing such a wacky, off-the-wall character as Sally on *3rd Rock from the Sun* would make such a glamorous look seem somewhat inappropriate on Kristen Johnston. Far from it. Kristen, like so many women, has different aspects of her personality that can be played up depending on mood and circumstance. And your hairstyle, like makeup and clothes, is like a prop to be used accordingly. So the more femme fatale the style, the more sexy you feel and act. Kristen, I must say, carries off the role superbly.

1 Shampoo, rinse, towel blot. Comb through conditioner, rinse, blot. (If necessary, use reconstructing conditioner on the hair about three times a week.)

2 Apply straightening gel with the heaviest application in back and on top of head, and more lightly around the face.

3 Spray styling spray around face and on the ends (places that will be ironed).

4 Part hair on one side and section from ear to ear across back of head. Pin to top of head.

5 Proceed with basic blow dry for straightening hair, followed by smoothing and polishing with round brush, turning the ends under. (Add a film of silicone to the ends for protection and smoothness.)

6 When hair is completely dry, add a film of creme groom.

7 From the part, going in both directions, divide the hair into forward and back sections.

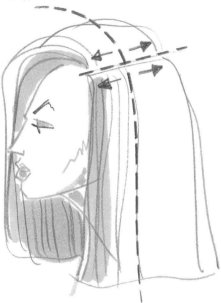

8 Starting with the front section of hair above the part, take small sections of hair and curl back from the hairline with the curling iron. Clip in place. (This can usually be done in four separate sections.) Note: If your hair is very straight, you can release the curl into a roller for a stronger set. Repeat on the shorter section (approximately three curls).

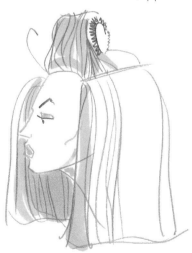

9 Release curls from clips and pull into wave with hands. Apply more groom if necessary.

10 Brush through curled and straightened hair together with finishing brush. If curl is too tight, blow it out with round brush and dryer until it relaxes. Finish off with a light spritz of holding spray.

Kristen Johnston, photographed by Don Flood

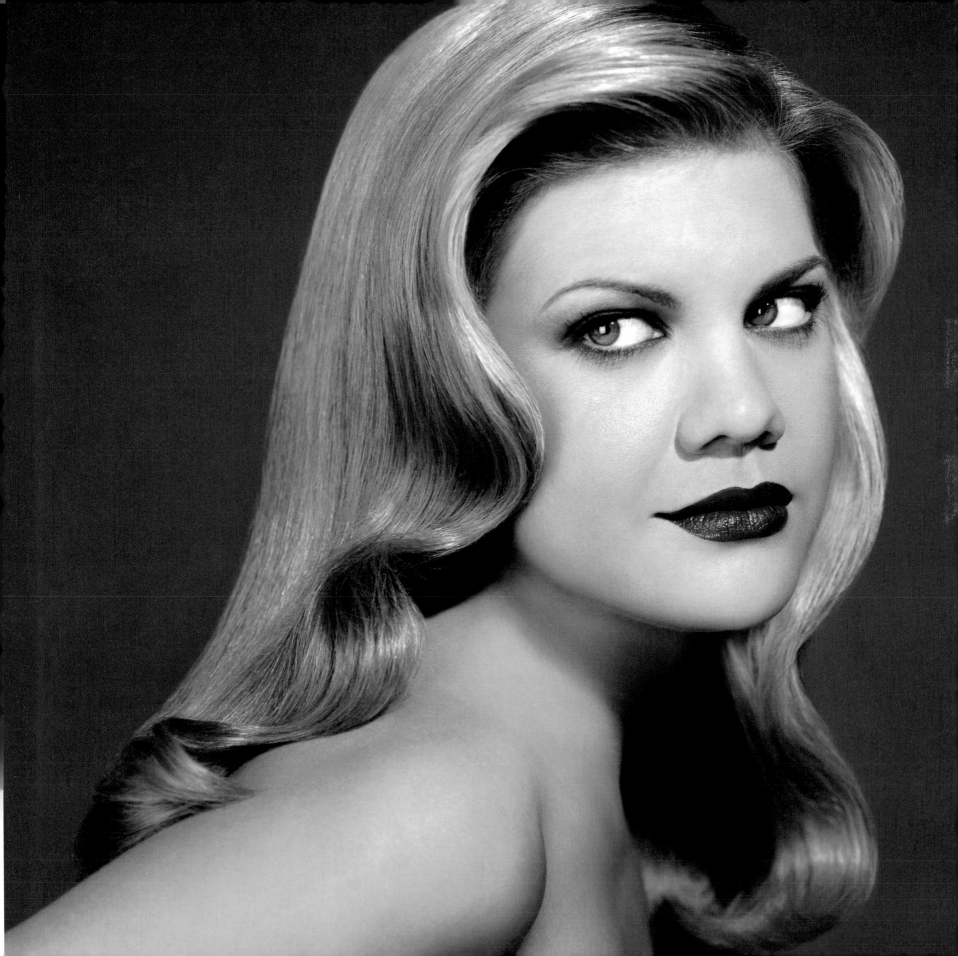

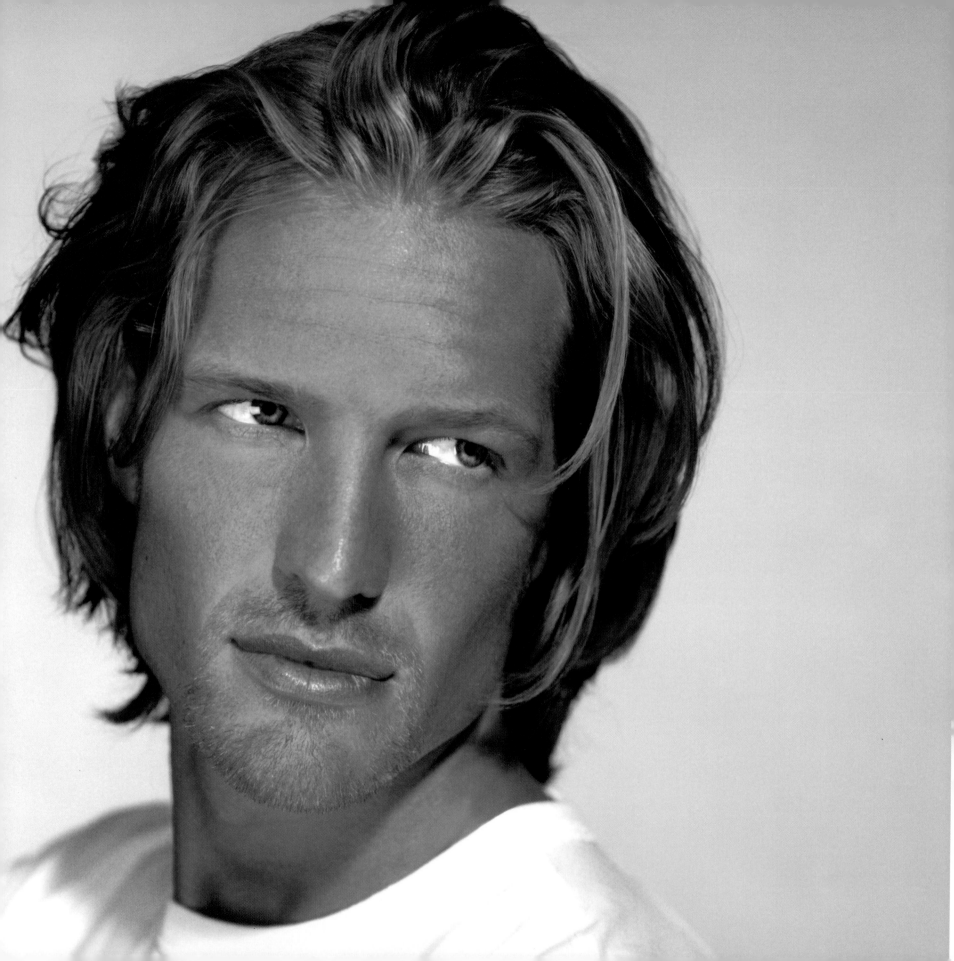

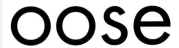

matt

hair type: thick, curly, and smooth
special process: none
cut: medium length, layers

tools
blow-drying brush • blow dryer with compressor
hard rubber fine-tooth comb

products
shampoo and conditioner (for dry, thick hair)
straightening gel • creme groom

I didn't want to leave you with the notion that men shouldn't or can't style their hair. The fact is many of them do if they have the opportunity or the inclination. Matt was the perfect subject to show you how a guy can take hair that is one texture and reconfigure it into another without feeling the least bit like he is overindulging himself in some sort of "beauty regimen."

To create this casual style, I basically used the same steps as outlined for Stephanie Seymour on page 100; however here there were two additional considerations.

One, the length of the hair is very important. As curly as it was to start, if Matt's hair were any shorter it would have been very difficult to grip it with a brush to straighten. And, as anyone with longer hair knows, the longer it is, the more its own weight will help to pull the curl out.

Second, creme groom was lightly applied to the hair to put a tiny bit of the curl back in and give it some movement. However, getting this soft waviness is only possible after you straighten the hair.

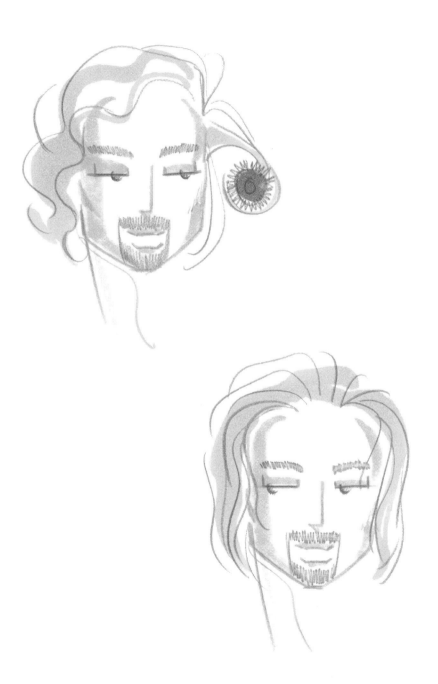

Matt King, photographed by Don Flood

The following individuals lent their considerable talents to making many of the images contained in this book as beautiful as they are.

Rumiko Hirose, *makeup artist:* cover, pages 25–27, 32–33, 44–45, 53–55, 58, 86, 89, 94, and 139.
Moyra Mulholland, *makeup artist:* pages 43, 47, 72–83, 85, 97, 101, 105, 109, and 135.
Susan McCarthy, *makeup artist:* pages 2–3, 24, 90, 93, and 110.
Carol Shaw, *makeup artist:* pages 116–117.
Lydia Snyder, *makeup artist:* pages 5 and 29.
Daphne Ballaso, *stylist:* pages 116–117 and 128.
Kelli Delaney, *stylist:* pages 43 and 105.
Jennifer Kyle, *stylist:* page 94.
Jennie Lopez, *stylist:* pages 72-83.
Robert Molnar, *stylist:* page 93.
Randi Packard, *stylist:* page 86.
Steven Amendola, *colorist:* cover, pages 5, 29, 54, 86, 94, 109, 135, and 141.

In addition, Cindy Crawford, photographed by Arthur Elgort on page 11, appears courtesy of *British Vogue.* Elizabeth Hurley, photographed by Torkil Gudnason on pages 14 and 114, appears courtesy of Estée Lauder. All Patrick Demarchelier photographs appear courtesy of Mr. Demarchelier and *Harper's Bazaar.* Brooke Shields on pages 122–23 appears courtesy of Mark Seliger, Drew Barrymore on page 127 appears courtesy of Wayne Maser, Halle Berry on page 142 appears courtesy of Gilles Bensimon, Revlon, and Tarlow Advertising. Melissa Brown on page 144 appears courtesy of Patric Shaw and *Allure.*

credits

On page 102: from top, Valentino and James Dean, courtesy of Kobal; Tab Hunter, courtesy of MacFadden/Corbis-Bettmann; Jeffrey Hunter, courtesy of Everett Collection. *On page 107*: from top, Veronica Lake, Elizabeth Taylor, Cher, and Farrah Fawcett, all courtesy of Kobal. *On page 111*: from top, Josephine Baker, Rita Hayworth, and Shirley Temple, all courtesy of Kobal; Brigitte Bardot, courtesy of Everett Collection. *On page 121*: from top, Louise Brooks and Audrey Hepburn, courtesy of Kobal; Mia Farrow, courtesy of Hulton Deutsch Collection/Corbis; Dorothy Hamill, courtesy of Everett Collection.

~ This photograph of Ashley Judd, taken by the incomparable Matthew Rolston, was part of a series of advertisements done for the design house of Carmen Marc Valvo. The intention, as you can gather from the image, was to re-create the mood of old Hollywood glamour portraiture. In this particular instance, Ashley's hair first had to be double processed to give it that "platinum blond" appearance. Once it was done, the texture of her hair easily allowed it to be styled into this amazing sculptural shape. Quite a transformation from her soft and short brunette look on page 20.

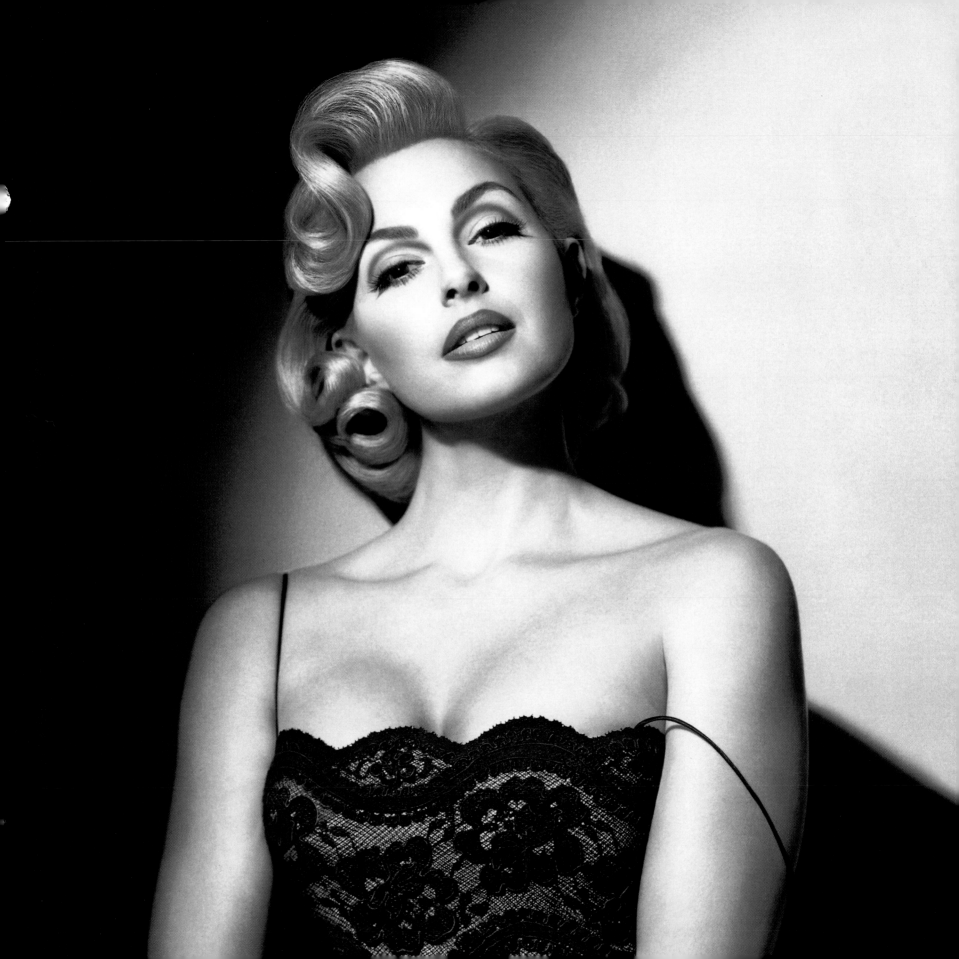

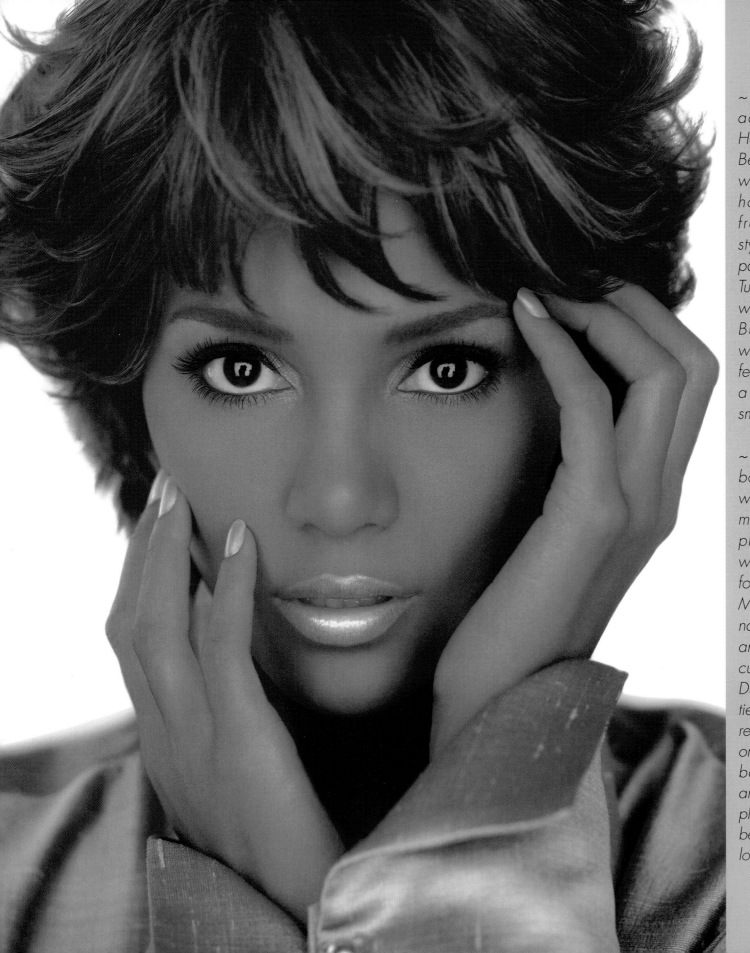

~ The looks you can achieve on fabulous Halle Berry are infinite. Believe me, not every woman can successfully hold her own going from such divergent styles as "Radiant" on page 110 to this Tina Turner–ish take, complete with softly spiked wig. But I've seen Halle wearing dozens of different coiffures and not a single one isn't a smash hit.

~ last page: I close the book with a beautiful windswept portrait of model Melissa Brown, photographed by the wonderful Patric Shaw for Allure. Judging from Melissa's previous incarnations, (pages 44–45 and 89) and this softly curled style (à la Faye Dunaway in the late sixties), you can see that it really is possible to take one texture (in this case, baby-fine blond hair) and successfully accomplish any one of a number of strikingly different looks. Go for it!

To Mom and Dad, Anne and Felix, thanks for all of your love and support. And to Mom, especially, thanks for the inspiration over the years. To my three brothers—Felix Jr., Steve, and Jerry—and two sisters—Lisa and Kim, thanks for trusting me with your tresses as I was learning the ropes. You were the perfect guinea pigs. And to my good friends Steven Amendola, Andy Armano, Paul Bellman, Leonard Calandra, Eva Chu, Rande Gerber, Nona Hendryx, Barbra Kurgan, Mark Ludwig, Moyra Mulholland, Carol Shaw, and Manabu Uno. I love you all.

To Maarten, thank you for keeping me grounded and centered during these many, many months. Having you in my life means everything to me. And to your parents, Paula and Pieter Van Der Sman, for making me a part of their family.

To Cindy Crawford, for being such a great friend and supporter all these years. You mean the world to me.

To everyone at Little, Brown & Company, from my amazingly enthusiastic editor Jennifer Josephy, to Linda Biagi, Matthew Ballast, Emily Fromm, Holly Wilkenson, Bryan Quible, Sarah Crichton, and many others, I am overwhelmed by your generosity and encouragement. All first-time authors should have it so good.

To my "mane" collaborator, Don Reuter, whose initial dearth of "hair-ticulture" proved one of the project's best assets, as we both learned to give each other what was needed to make this book happen, making it into everything I wanted it to be and then some.

To my unflagging agent, Jed Root, and his entire staff, including Kellie O'Bosky, Patrick O'Leary, Katie Yu, Laura Ball, Chris O'Leary, Leo Victoria, and Joanne Salt-Arborio, over the past few months and throughout the years I appreciate your attention and guidance. To Marcy Engleman, for coming through for me like a true champion. To Jami and Klaus Heidegger, Cammie Burns, and Jason Schell of Kiehl's, I don't know what I would have done without you.

To Don Flood, Nicolai Grosell, Troy Word, Neal Barr, and Jay Zukerkorn, for contributing their amazing photographic talents and unbelievable generosity with their time and work. Gentlemen, I am forever grateful. And to Pascal Dangin, for putting just the right amount of the extraordinary into already superlative work. Genius.

To the subjects of *The Mane Thing,* who took time from their busy schedules to sit for a gathering of magnificent portraits, including Emme Aronson, Halle Berry, Melissa Brown, Jenny Brunt, Taren Cunningham, Heather Dillon, Karen "Duff" Duffy, Kashanna Evans, John Francis, Daisy Fuentes, Charlie Goring, A. J. Hammer, Angie Hsu, Kristen Johnston, Kidada Jones, Rashida Jones, James King, Matt King, Peggy Lipton, Amanda Moore, Oluchi, Stephanie Seymour, Rachel Shane, and Ella Thomas.

And to the following individuals who contributed their considerable talent, artistry, and work, including Steven Amendola, Michel Arnaud, Daphne Ballaso, Gilles Bensimon, Leilani Bishop, Naomi Campbell, Christina Cruze, Kelli Delaney, Patrick Demarchelier, Sante D'Orazio, Arthur Elgort, Janine Giddings, Shalom Harlow, Salma Hayek, Rumiko Hirose, George Holz, Marc Hom, Linda Hop, Kirsty Hume, Ashley Judd, Jennifer Kyle, Jennie Lopez, Wayne Maser, Susan McCarthy, Robert Molnar, Phoebe O'Brien, Randi Packard, Jaime Rishar, Matthew Rolston,

Isabella Rossellini, Francesco Scavullo, Mark Seliger, Carol Shaw, Patric Shaw, Lydia Snyder, Niki Taylor, Christy Turlington, and Amber Valetta.

I would also like to thank the following individuals and organizations for all their help in putting this book together, and for their continued support over the years: Almay, ARGroup, Amy Astley, Kevyn Aucoin, Maria Avitable, Ally B., Sheril Bailey, Drew Barrymore, Alisa Belletini, Emily Bennett-Wheeler, Chris Bishop and Bishop Studio, Alexis Borges, Betsy Boudreaux, Christie Brinkley, Terry Brogan, Ron Byland, David Cameron, Carmen Marc Valvo, John Carrasco, Paul Cavaco, Fabio Chizzola, Gregg Christensen, Cindy and Peter Cirlin, Clairol, Carol Clark, Company, Michel Comte, Chris Connors, Nick Constantinesco, Fran Cooper, Peter Coppola, Bob Cosenza of the Kobal Collection, Norman Curry of Corbis-Bettmann, Fran Curtis, Helene Curtis, Danilo, Alex Davis, Geena Davis, DDBNeedham Chicago, Joanne DeCarlo, Kim Delaney, Meryl Delierre of the Everett Collection, John Dellaria, Tom Dey, Peg Donegan, Marianne Dougherty, Drive-In Studio, Brian Dubin, Ruth Eagleton-Grocott, Elite, Annee Elliott, Robert Erdmann, Fulvia Farolfi, Anne Fisher, Michael Flutie, Eric Gabriel, Alessia Glaviano, Randy Gonzalez, Tonne Goodman, Grey Advertising, Desiree Gruber, Paul Guayante, Torkil Gudnason, Neil Hamel, Jennifer Harrison, Lynn Hirschberg, Christophe Hitz, Marianne Houtenbos, Elizabeth Hurley, Anjelica Huston, IMG, Industria Superstudio, Kathy Ireland, Anne Marie Iverson, Lisa Jacobsen, JGK, Jim Johnson, Karen Johnson, Donna Karan,

acknowledgments

Christine Karl, Corinne Karr, Sonia Kashuk, Kirsten Kenney, Stella Kleinrock, Dan Klores, Pat Koleser, Becca Kovacik, Kevin Krier, Aerin Lauder, Estée Lauder, Tracy LeBrecque-Davis, Jacqui Lefton, Freddie Leiba, Denise Leong, Gideon Lewin, Lifetime, Mia Lolordo, L'Oréal, Jean Louis, Julia Louis-Dreyfus, Courtney Love, John Lum of Comzone, Andrew MacPherson, Delia Martinez, Wendell Maruyama, Brett McCartney, Mary McConnell, Martha McCully, Ray McKigney, Steven Meisel, Bill Melamed, Polly Mellen, Laura Mercier, Joyce Mills, Jeff Moore, William Morris, Helen Murray, Ken Nahoum, Mayumi Nakashima, Francois Nars, Missie Neville, Helmut Newton, Next, Dewey Nicks, Serge Normand, Caroline Noseworthy, Omar, Oribe, Dick Page, Pantene, Pauline's, Kristen Perrotta, Philips, Jason Phillips, Rosemary Prodo, Charles Purvis, Jean Renard, Revlon, Mia Ricchiuti, Herb Ritts, Andrea Robinson, Rogers & Cowan, RSA, Winona Ryder, Elisa Santisi, Vidal Sassoon, Terry-Jo Shahidi, Shear World, Brooke Shields, Matthew Shields, Smashbox Studio, Solano, Jennifer Steffancin, Studio One, Tarlow Advertising, Michelle Thomas, J. Walter Thompson, Michael Thompson, Liz Tilberus, Alexis Tolbert, Twist Productions, Betsy Uhrig, David Vallin, Kimberly Wang, Mary Warner, Ginny Washburn, Albert Watson, Linda Wells, Neal Werner, David White, Michael Whitman of Metropolis, and Wolf-Kasteler.

Finally, I want to acknowledge all the magazines, editors, makeup artists, stylists, advertising agencies, cosmetic and hair-care companies, directors, models, celebrities, agents, bookers, assistants, and fellow hairstylists whom I have had the pleasure of knowing (and working with) over these many years. This is truly a wonderful business to be a part of, and I thank you all.

Halle Berry, photographed by Gilles Bensimon for Revlon